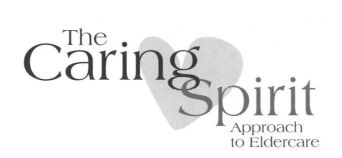

The Caring Spirit

Approach
to Eldercare

The Caring Spirit

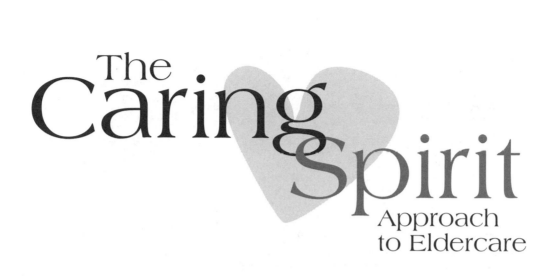

Approach to Eldercare

A Training Guide for
Professionals and Families

by

Nancy L. Kriseman, M.S.W., L.C.S.W.

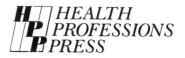

HEALTH
PROFESSIONS
PRESS

Baltimore • London • Sydney

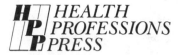

Health Professions Press
Post Office Box 10624
Baltimore, Maryland 21285-0624

www.healthpropress.com

Typeset by Erin Geoghegan.
Manufactured in the United States of America by
Versa Press, Inc., East Peoria, Illinois.

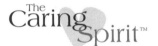

The Caring Spirit™ is a trademark owned by Nancy L. Kriseman.
For information, contact www.nancykriseman.com or nancykriseman@comcast.net.

Library of Congress Cataloging-in-Publication Data
Kriseman, Nancy L.
  The caring spirit approach to eldercare : a training guide for professionals and families / by Nancy L. Kriseman.
     p. ; cm.
  Includes bibliographical references.
  ISBN 1-932529-06-3
  1. Older people--Care. 2. Older people--Services for. 3. Caregivers.
  [DNLM: 1. Health Services for the Aged. 2. Family Relations. 3. Professional-Patient Relations. 4. Spirituality. WT 31 K92c 2005] I. Title.
  RA564.8.K75 2005
  362'.0425'0846--dc22
                              2005007858

British Library Cataloguing in Publication data are available from the British Library.

Contents

This book is dedicated to my parents, who inspired
much of this work, along with all the families
who have touched my spirit over the years.

Acknowledgments

I wish to extend my thanks to ARC (Atlanta Regional Commission) for granting the funding to create and write some of the training modules appearing in *The Caring Spirit Approach to Eldercare*. The ARC also provided partial funding for piloting this training program in a nursing home. I appreciate the confidence demonstrated in this care philosophy by the ARC's support of this program.

I also wish to thank the Georgia Long-term Care Ombudsman Program and the Georgia Department of Human Resources' Division of Aging Services (Area Agencies on Aging) for helping to fund the pilot program for *The Caring Spirit* training.

I am especially indebted to all the wonderful people who helped me with the development of the initial ten training modules, including helping to research books and articles, evaluate measurement scales, and read and edit the manuscript: Eve Levine, L.C.S.W.; Stephanie Roach, L.C.S.W.; Edie Cohen; Jennifer Norton; Pat Rich; Sharon Smith; Tracy Stetler; Vicki Patterson, Ph.D.; and Mary Ball, Ph.D.

My very special thanks to Kerry Kriseman, who edited the initial ten training modules with a "caring heart" and to Stephanie Roach, L.C.S.W., my dear friend and colleague who edited the entire manuscript with a true "caring spirit." Also to Mary Magnus, Director of Publications for Health Professions Press, for her continued support and encouragement, and for keeping my spirit alive throughout the birthing of this book. She is a true "caring spirit." And finally, thanks to Cynthia, who has listened endlessly to my trials and tribulations while writing this book, offered wise suggestions, and supported me throughout. She is "my caring spirit."

Foreword

It is one of the ironies of our time that the further medical technology advances, the greater the need for the caring spirit in the work we do. I remember being given a small, red, hardcover book when I was in my final year of medical school. It did not contain the latest medications and their dosages, nor did it include a list of lab values and their normal ranges. Instead, its pages held the wisdom of a turn-of-the-century physician. The title, *The Care of the Patient,* said it all. It could easily be read in one sitting. The words that have stayed with me all these years, and that still remind me of the most important part of being a physician, are as true as the sky: "The secret to caring for the patient is caring for the patient." In other words, we must never lose sight of the fundamentally human nature of caring. Technology is a fine thing. It saves lives, it limits suffering, but it is not care and should never be offered as a substitute for caring.

This realization leads to the deeper question: Is a caring approach to those who are ill an inborn trait that comes in abundance to some and hardly at all to others? Or, is the *spirit of caring* something that can be learned, something that can be taught, something that can be caught? These questions bedevil the admissions committees at medical and nursing schools. In hospitals and nursing homes, directors of nursing peer into the eyes of those they hire, looking for the caring spirit. It is probably best to straddle this fence. Certainly some people arrive at the doorstep of health care organizations ready, willing, and able to embrace the work of caring, while many others have much less inborn talent in this area. The nature of the many regular people (born without the Mother Teresa gene) calls out to us all. We must, by every means possible, expand our ability to reach them and to teach them the caring spirit. This was the intention behind the distribution of that little red book to the medical students of my class so many years ago.

Fortunately for us all, Nancy Kriseman goes far beyond the musings of a long-dead physician and offers us concrete advice about how to be caring, including specific steps we can take to innoculate those around us with *the caring spirit.* I have seen many books that suggest actions that might be successful. Ms. Kriseman has done us all a great favor by rigorously testing her concepts in practice and over time before writing her book. It takes little to tell others what *ought* to work; it takes much to show others what *does* work. Her dedication to the latter makes this book very sweet indeed.

This book should be kept within easy reach because it can help you help others enter into and be enriched by all that genuine caring has to offer. This is a precious gift, perhaps the most precious of all that can be given. And received.

William H. Thomas, M.D.
Founder, The Eden Alternative
Summer Hill, New York

Preface

Do all the good you can
By all the means you can
In all the ways you can
In all the places you can
To all the people you can
As long as you can
—John Wesley

I am a licensed geriatric clinical social worker who has been working with elders and the staff who care for them since 1982. I am also the daughter of a mother with Alzheimer's disease. At the time this book is published, my mother will have been living in a nursing home for 9 years.

Textbooks, classrooms, and training teach those of us working in long-term care to be aware of our elders' physical, emotional, and even intellectual needs, but nothing as yet prepares us for how to *care* for our elders in the context of what is perhaps the most spiritual period of their lives.

Throughout my career, and from my firsthand experience with my mother, I have been privileged to witness the challenges and triumphs of eldercare from the perspective of both the caregiver and the recipient. What I have learned is that this work is hard and that the intention of those doing it is often positive. I also have observed that the life adjustment for elders at this stage is profound.

In working with direct care staff and other professionals who care for elders, I have come to respect and appreciate the difficult work they do. What has reinforced my professional insights has been spending time with my mother as she lived out her last years with Alzheimer's disease in a nursing home. Spending significant time with my mother week after week revealed how differently she responded to staff members who approached her in a more humanistic way. When staff members attempted to reach out to her spirit and soul instead of relating to her as just another Alzheimer's disease patient, mechanically providing only the ADL (activities of daily living) care she needed, I noticed a big difference in how she responded to them. When the staff members approached my mother from their hearts, with compassion, they connected to her spirit and soul. As a result, my mother was calmer, less agitated, and more receptive to the care they provided for her.

For years I had noticed that something *significant* was missing from our long-term care training, but it took experiences like these to discern what it was. I came to believe that we must provide care staff and families with the resources to connect to themselves in more spiritually meaningful ways. I also came to believe that helping elders *finish well* requires environments that affirm spiritual connections.

The Caring Spirit approach that I have developed and share in this training guide offers staff, families, and professionals who work with and care for elders a way to recognize and enhance the spiritual lives of elders, to care for them from a spiritual place. This innovative training program places high regard on the staff members who work with elders, helping them to view their work as sacred. When elders are viewed as full human beings, the potential emerges for staff members and elders to enrich each others' lives and experience a more caring community in which to live and work. Families and elders also have the potential to develop a more meaningful connection to one another at the end of life. Promoting this change is the mission of *The Caring Spirit Approach to Eldercare: A Training Guide for Professionals and Families.*

It is my hope that readers will come away from this book thinking differently about the later stage of life and wanting to use *The Caring Spirit*™ approach as a way to change the culture in long-term care. I also hope that all who participate in this program, either as trainers or as participants, will enjoy *The Caring Spirit* training modules and recognize the impact they could have on staff, families, elders, and all professionals who work with elders.

Blessings to you and may you hold onto *the caring spirit* in all aspects of your life!

Nancy L. Kriseman, M.S.W, L.C.S.W.
www.nancykriseman.com

How to Use this Book and Training Program

The Caring Spirit™ approach provides a unique perspective on how professional and family caregivers who care for elders can use spiritual values as the focus for caring. *The Caring Spirit* takes caring to a deeper level, recognizing the true meaning of *caring* and the ethics involved in providing compassionate care. *The Caring Spirit* helps to foster a mutually positive experience between elders and the professional and family caregivers who provide their care.

FOR PROFESSIONALS

The Caring Spirit training modules were created to help the members of a professional care staff connect to their work and to themselves in more spiritually meaningful ways. Using *The Caring Spirit* philosophy can help professionals experience their work as sacred. The training modules also present opportunities for staff members to learn different ways to take care of themselves and to recognize the challenges of their jobs.

FOR FAMILIES

Several of *The Caring Spirit* training modules were created to help family members learn to cope more effectively with the challenges they face when caring for elder family members. In addition, *The Caring Spirit* philosophy helps family caregivers recognize the importance of taking better care of themselves. They receive helpful tips and guidance for improved self care.

HOW TO IMPLEMENT THE TRAINING MODULES

Each chapter of this book contains the following material:

- An explanation of the principles behind the lessons in that chapter's training module

- A complete training module, with step-by-step instructions for trainers about how to introduce the training session, lead a warm-up exercise and a core exercise, and close the training session

- All participant handouts

- All trainer handouts

- A participant evaluation form for the training session

Before beginning to work with this material, trainers will want to read the Introduction to this book, which explains why *The Caring Spirit* approach was created and provides a short description of each training module. Also, the background information presented in the beginning of each chapter provides insight into each topic covered in the modules.

Trainers should be aware of several points about the training modules and exercises:

- Each training module is interactive, providing participants with the opportunity to participate in engaging exercises that may involve discussions, experiential activities, or short games. These interactive exercises give participants a unique insight into what they are learning.

- Participants may be asked to discuss sensitive subjects during the training sessions. It is important, therefore, to establish a trusting and comfortable learning environment during these trainings (see Sensitivity of the Training Material below).

- Some of the exercises in the modules require participants to bring items such as music, food, pictures, or poetry to the training sessions. The trainer needs to remind participants of any items they need to bring to the next session.

- Quotes appear in the chapter text and training modules that can be used as teaching tools. Some of the quotes are already incorporated into the exercises, but the trainer can also select some of the other quotes to incorporate into the training.

- Many of the modules have handouts for the interactive exercises. It is important for the trainer to review the handouts before each session and ensure that enough copies are available for all participants.

- Some of the interactive exercises have instructions that the trainer should read carefully prior to conducting the training session so that he or she is comfortable explaining the exercise to the participants.

Following are several additional important points for trainers:

- One week prior to starting *The Caring Spirit* training, the trainer should introduce this unique, spirituality-based training program to the participants. A handout for trainers to give to participants that summarizes the program is provided at the end of this section.

- Because each session is only an hour-and-a-half long and the training completely fills this time, the trainer needs to emphasize the importance of promptness in attendance at the training sessions. It is recommended that guidelines be implemented to minimize tardiness.

- The trainer should inform participants that evaluation forms must be completed at the conclusion of each session. It is helpful to explain the importance of these evaluations, for example that they provide an opportunity for reflection on what has been learned and ensure that what participants are learning is helpful to them. The evaluations also provide a way for participants to suggest ideas or present thoughts and feelings they did not feel free to express during training. Finally, they inform the trainer about whether the trainer's approach is understandable, helpful, and interesting. The trainer should remind participants not to worry about spelling and grammar. And if anyone is not comfortable with writing, the trainer can assist him or her.

- The trainer will want to close each training session by thanking staff or family members for participating in this unique training opportunity and by previewing the upcoming session.

- At the end of the training program, after all the sessions are completed, the trainer should provide an opportunity for all participants to share something positive that they gained from being a part of the training program.

SENSITIVITY OF THE TRAINING MATERIAL

Some of *The Caring Spirit* training modules contain sensitive material that may elicit a range of emotions and feelings from the participants. It is imperative for the trainer to set a tone for the training that allows participants to feel safe and comfortable sharing their feelings. The trainer should stress to staff members that, because they are discussing sensitive topics, the sessions are to be treated as strictly confidential and comments are to be kept between participants only.

The following comments have been made by former participants and will give the trainer insight into how sensitive this material can be for some participants:

"It reinforced thoughts, feelings and beliefs I already possessed and introduced me to new ways of thinking about my feelings."

"It was helpful in allowing me to get in touch with my inner self."

"I realize about myself that I need to be thankful for my life and the people around. It also helps me when I was down about my best friend who had died."

"I realized how important it is to not be afraid to express myself and my feelings."

"It taught me about other people's feelings aside from my own, and it made me understand the meaning of loving and caring…"

"I realized that many times I work and my spirit is not with me; I feel bad about that."

"This training let us openly express ourselves."

"I learned more about my emotions and my well-being."

"It gave us a chance to talk about spirituality, which is not normally talked about and which is important to our well being."

Introduction

"I contend, however, that all things being equal,
we will work harder and more effectively for people
we like. And we will like them in direct proportion
to how they make us feel."
James Kouzes & Barry Posner, from *Credibility*

The Caring Spirit training program was developed as a result of several concerns:

1. The low staff morale and high turnover prevalent in long-term care settings and how these factors affect care.

2. The lack of training programs available to help family caregivers process their feelings about caregiving.

3. The lack of training available to provide families and professionals with spiritual resources to help them cope with the inevitable stresses of caregiving.

MEETING CARE STAFF NEEDS

When addressing the concern of low staff morale and high turnover in long-term care settings, research reveals a discrepancy between how staff members behaved in their jobs and what they reported as their reasons for choosing the work they did. Staff members seemed unhappy and unmotivated in their jobs, and they demonstrated low morale. Yet when asked in training sessions why they chose the work they did, staff members usually responded with very positive comments, such as these collected during the many years I have provided training to long-term care professionals:

"I love older people."

"My mama always told me I would care for people who needed my help."

"My grandmother was such an inspiration to me; I want to give back what she taught me."

"Older people have wonderful stories to tell."

"I like being with older people because they appreciate what you do for them."

"I know they can't care for themselves and I want to help them."

"They make me laugh."

"They feel like family to me."

Thus, a gap appears to exist between job satisfaction and people's original purpose for taking the job. This raises two questions:

- Why do staff members lose *spirit* toward the elders and their work?

- Why is there such a wide gap between job satisfaction and a person's original purpose for taking the job?

Understanding Training Approaches for Staff

In an effort to answer these questions, I researched some of the newer staff training programs to see whether *different* approaches to training were being explored, and if the training being conducted was sensitive to the eldercare challenges that staff face when providing care. Several training paradigms—the Best Friends approach, the Wellspring model, and the Better Life philosophy of Apple Health Care—seemed to be more innovative in their thinking about eldercare and training. These programs focused on the critical issues of retention and turnover, staff morale, and poor work performance. They recognized the need to provide a different approach to training. They also addressed important training issues that have formerly been overlooked. For example, they have

- Reexamined the *content* of the training provided, making sure it helps the staff acquire the skills needed to provide the best care to elders

- Stressed the importance of having content that is appropriate to the education level of the staff

- Focused on the need to provide more *interactive* training for the staff

- Highlighted the need for commitment from the administration to train all staff and encourage a learning community

- Suggested that consistent supervision and follow-up with staff members is necessary to reinforce what is being learned and to provide opportunities for staff members to feel appreciated for their efforts

- Acknowledged that for staff members to accomplish their jobs, they need to have the necessary tools, and these tools need to be easily accessible

- Promoted creating a learning environment that is less distracting and more conducive to learning

Despite these positive changes offered by the new paradigms, a key component still was missing. The training programs did not focus on how staff members *felt* about their work or how they could be helped to feel more *spirited* in their work.

One of the distinguishing features and key components of *The Caring Spirit* training program is the notion that staff members need training that includes helping them *connect to their spirits* and develop more *caring attitudes* toward themselves and the elders for whom they care.

The Caring Spirit training program provides a foundation for orienting staff to an agency's philosophy of care. It emphasizes an ethical approach to care and provides a framework for helping staff recognize the value of their work. In addition, it sets the stage for all other training offered by a facility. If staff can maintain a *caring spirit* attitude toward their work and their peers, and if future staff training can emphasize *The Caring Spirit* philosophy, then turnover could be reduced and job satisfaction enhanced.

MEETING FAMILY CAREGIVER NEEDS

Another reason behind the creation of *The Caring Spirit* training program was the lack of training programs for family caregivers, especially any with a focus on helping them become more familiar with their feelings about caregiving and learn how to care for themselves. A plethora of research indicates that caregiving is stressful and can cause depression and other illnesses. Few training programs, however, address how to help families find positive and spiritual ways to cope with stress and take better care of their minds, bodies and spirits.

Following are some of the responses family members provided when asked in various training sessions why they do not take care of themselves:

- They were not willing to ask for support and help. They felt that there were not enough available supports and resources, or they did not know how to access them.

- They felt it was their job to be the caregiver.

- They were too overwhelmed to take care of themselves or felt they did not have time.

- They were in denial that they were stressed and tired.

- They did not know how to communicate their needs.

- They did not want to bother anyone and felt it was their responsibility (spouses/partners particularly felt this way).

- They felt powerless or paralyzed and did not even know where to begin.

Clearly a gap exists between recognizing that family caregivers are stressed and depressed and providing ways to help them cope. It raises several questions:

- What type of training might best address the caregivers' concerns?

- What kinds of approaches might lead to more effective coping strategies for these family members?

- Why isn't a spiritual approach to caring for oneself being promoted with family caregivers?

WHERE DO PROFESSIONALS' AND FAMILY CAREGIVERS' NEEDS OVERLAP?

In reviewing current research around the concept of care, it became apparent that *care* and *spirituality* were related. It also became clear that both professional and family caregivers could benefit from training with a spiritual approach. It would help both types of caregivers find additional healthy solutions to coping with the demands of caregiving. *The Caring Spirit* training program, therefore, attempts to revitalize the *spirit* of caregivers and help them get in touch with their hearts and souls. Spiritual values and the ethics surrounding caring are particularly emphasized. I have come to believe that if a spiritual approach to training is utilized, then training and caregiving have the potential to generate new meaning and produce more effective outcomes.

CREATING A CULTURE OF CARING IN TRAINING

"[Caring] is an expression of loving.
It's how loving makes itself known."
John Morton, from *The Blessings Already Are*

As advances in medicine enable people to live longer, society will be caring for more elders than ever before. As the start of the 21st century unfolds, at least 20 percent of the population will be 65 years old and older, and the fastest-growing segment of the population is already the 85-and-older age group. The challenge, then, is how to care for this ever-increasing population so that elders are truly cared for and about and not just kept alive.

In their book *Rethinking Alzheimer's Care*, authors, Fazio, Seman, and Stansell attempted to define what *caring for* elders truly means. They presented several noteworthy concepts, which are prefaced with the following questions:

- What does it mean to *care* for someone?

- What does *caring about or for* others mean to the person providing the care?

- How can someone care for someone else in a way that does not make him or her feel like an object?

- How does caring for someone help him or her?

- How does *caring* differ from *providing care*?

- What does it mean to care for someone's own family or friends, and for one-self?

The authors believe that the changes occurring in longevity rates and in health care will require staff who work with elders to have a clearer philosophy of caring that will support understanding how to preserve a caring approach. While these authors were mainly addressing professional caregivers, the same issues need to be addressed with family caregivers as well.

In conclusion, Fazio, et al., suggested guidelines for considering caring in a different way, stating that

- Caring helps support the self-esteem of the elder

- Caring helps diminish anxiety and fear

- Caring helps the elder feel safe, physically and emotionally

- Caring lets the person know he or she is important and valued

- Caring increases the likelihood of successful completion of tasks that are needed for the elder

- Caring provides the staff with a feeling of satisfaction and gratification

From these guidelines, it can be concluded that caring is one of the ways in which people manifest their spiritual selves in the world. Reflecting on caring in that way, several additional guidelines could be added to those listed above:

- Caring is a spiritual act. When staff members, families, and elders care for each other, it can help them feel more deeply connected to themselves and to one another.

- Caring is an act of loving kindness that places two people in a sacred space together.

- Caring requires considering the spirit of the person as well as the mind and body.

- Caring requires bringing our spiritual values to the caregiving process.

Expecting quality of care for our elders requires recognizing the importance of creating a *culture of caring* for those who live and work in long-term care settings. Creating a culture of caring requires two components:

1. Management must ensure that all who live and work in long-term care environments are treated with respect, compassion, and caring.

2. Staff members must be appreciated and valued.

We cannot expect caregivers to provide quality care to elders if we do not value their work and provide them with the training and tools they need to conduct their jobs with integrity and caring. My approach to creating a culture of caring emphasizes compassionate values, a solid sense of ethics, and continued recognition of the sacredness of the end of life. *The Caring Spirit* philosophy provides the spiritual groundwork needed to create such a culture of caring in long-term care settings.

Questions to Ponder When Taking a Spiritual Approach to Training with Professionals and Families

The questions below set the stage for thinking about how a *spiritual* approach to training changes the context of the training for professionals and families.

Questions for Professionals

1. **How does this training program nurture the spirits and souls of the staff so they in turn can nurture the spirits and souls of the elders?**

   - Are staff members provided with ways to exhibit their strengths?

   - Are there opportunities for staff members to share their spiritual sides?

   - Are staff members empowered to tap into their spirituality to help them through the more difficult situations?

   - Are staff members provided with the "compassionate tools" they need to work in a caring way with our elders?

   - Are staff members shown that their knowledge and experience is valued?

   - What opportunities are provided for staff members to *know* one another?

   - Are staff members honored and respected in ways they can reciprocate with the elders?

   - What opportunities are provided for the staff to have a more spiritual environment in which to work?

   - How is a *culture of caring* created and maintained in the work environment?

2. **How do training programs encourage staff to *know* the elders for whom they care?**

   - Are staff members asked in training exercises to share information and stories about the elders in their care?

   - Are staff members provided with good background information about every elder for whom they are expected to provide care?

   - Are staff members given enough time to provide individualized care to residents in their care?

   - Are staff members given information about the religious or cultural backgrounds of elders in their care?

Once these questions are addressed, staff can begin receiving the best possible training in the most spiritual way.

Questions for Families

1. **How does this training program nurture the spirits and souls of family caregivers so they in turn can nurture the spirits and souls of their loved ones?**

   - Are there opportunities for family caregivers to recognize their spiritual sides?

   - Are families empowered to lean on their spirituality to help them through difficult situations?

   - Are family caregivers encouraged to nurture themselves? Are they provided with the skills needed to do so?

   - Are they taught to recognize how stress and depression can be indicators that their spirits are not being nurtured?

   - Are family caregivers taught spiritual approaches to coping with stress in addition to other traditional approaches?

Once these questions are addressed, it is likely that more effective coping skills can be available for family caregivers. By participating in *The Caring Spirit* program, family caregivers will have the opportunity to find comfort in a spiritual approach to caring for themselves while they are caring for their loved ones.

OVERVIEW OF *THE CARING SPIRIT* TRAINING PROGRAM FOR PROFESSIONAL STAFF

The objectives of *The Caring Spirit* training program for professionals are

- To promote a more positive culture within a facility's care community

- To encourage a more compassionate, spiritual approach to caring for elders

- To improve staff morale

- To promote more positive feelings and job satisfaction

The Caring Spirit training program for professionals contains ten interactive training modules designed to meet these objectives. Together, the modules also accomplish these additional tasks:

- Encourage team building.

- Help build a bond of trust among participants.

- Help participants become more aware of their inner selves.

- Help participants recognize their talents and skills.

- Generate more positive communication among participants, with the goal of building a *culture of caring* among all staff members and elders.

- Help participants recognize when their own spirits are in jeopardy so they can take a more spiritual approach to providing better care for themselves.

Each module is an hour-and-a-half in length and was created to be a stand-alone session. Each module builds upon the others, however, and it is recommended that participants commit to attending all ten sessions.

Module One: Understanding Spirituality and Your Spiritual Self

The focus of this training module is to open the pathways for participants to explore what spirituality means to them and to others. They will explore ways to tap into their own spiritual selves. In addition, they will learn how being spiritual can lead to a different way of caring for themselves and for the elders with whom they work.

Module Two: Creating a Spiritual Work Environment

The focus here is on how to create a more spiritual work environment, exploring what *home* means to participants and to the elders in their care. Participants also develop a definition of the concept of a *culture of caring*, exploring the importance of having a caring culture in which to live and work.

Module Three: Why Working in Eldercare Is a Blessing

Working through this module helps participants appreciate the work they do and gain a better understanding of why they do this kind of work. They explore why working with elders is a *blessing*. Participants also examine the many ways in which they are *blessed* to work with each other and how it is a privilege to help elders *finish well*. As participants become more aware of the many blessings in their lives, they are more apt to feel the abundance they gain from their jobs.

Module Four: How Inspiration Affects
Staff Members and Those for Whom They Care

Inspiration helps motivate staff members and reinforces the value of their work. This training module helps them identify who has inspired them in their lives and what inspiration means to them. It helps them answer the questions, "What inspires me to work with elders?" and "How can we inspire each other?"

Module Five: Spiritual Approaches to Caring for Elders

Caring for elders at the end of their lives is challenging but can also be seen as *sacred*. Understanding how to approach elders in a more spiritual way can transform the caregiving experience. The following issues are explored in this module:

- How professionals can be more spiritual in their approach to care

- How a spiritual approach to care differs from a more traditional approach

- How taking a more spiritual approach to caring affects the way caregivers feel about themselves and the elders for whom they care

Module Six: How Staff Members Can Find Support within the Work They Do

This training module takes participants on a journey to find their inner strengths and additional ways to help them care for elders. Participants will also explore external sources of strength. They will consider how the work they do is angel-like.

Module Seven: Spiritual Ways to Cope with Stress

Through this training module participants acknowledge how stressful their jobs can be. They learn some less traditional ways to cope with stress, including spiritual coping tools introduced through various exercises that allow participants to practice these different ways to cope with stress. Participants can come to see stress as an opportunity for growth and change.

Module Eight: Communicating from the Heart

In this training module, participants find the *path to their hearts*. They learn the concept of *spiritual listening* and recognize how it can help them communicate more successfully with the elders for whom they care. Participants will learn about barriers that interfere with communicating from the heart, as well as some alternative ways to communicate in their personal and work lives.

Module Nine: Staying Connected Through Rituals

Connecting to the past and to the present can often be accomplished by exploring rituals. This training module looks at the role participants' own family rituals play in their relationships at work and in their day-to-day activities. Participants will have a better understanding of why it is important to preserve the rituals of the elders in their care.

Module Ten: Taking Care of Our Own Spirits

This module allows participants to explore why they tend not to take adequate care of themselves and how this impacts their work lives. They learn the concept of being *self-full* along with the symptoms of burnout. Finally, participants learn ways to take care of themselves in a more *caring spirit* way.

OVERVIEW OF *THE CARING SPIRIT* TRAINING PROGRAM FOR FAMILY CAREGIVERS

The objectives of *The Caring Spirit* training program for family caregivers are:

- To promote a more compassionate understanding of the role of the family caregiver

- To encourage family caregivers to take better care of their own spirits by using spiritual coping tools

- To help family members understand both the grieving process and the role changes that occur when caring for a loved one

The Caring Spirit training program for family caregivers meets these objectives in four interactive training modules. The specific purpose of each module varies, but all are designed to accomplish the following tasks:

- Encourage participants to share their feelings and concerns.

- Help build a bond of trust among participants.

- Help participants recognize their shared concerns and challenges.

- Help participants recognize when their own spirits are in jeopardy so they can take a more spiritual approach to providing better care for themselves.

Each module is an hour-and-a-half in length and was created to be a stand-alone session. Each module builds upon the others, however, and it is recommended that participants commit to participating in all four sessions.

Module Eleven: Why a Spiritual Approach to Caring Matters

The focus of this training module is to help families learn additional ways to cope with the caregiving experience. They will have the opportunity to explore what their spirituality means to them and to their loved ones. They will learn how to tap into their own spiritual sides and gain a clearer understanding of how being spiritual can lead to a different way of caring for themselves and their loved ones.

Module Twelve: Helping Families Connect from the Heart

This training module helps participants find the path to their hearts. They will explore how communicating from their hearts can help them communicate with their loved ones in a deeper way, and how communicating solely from the "head" blocks them from their heart and from the ways of the heart. Participants will discuss barriers to communicating from the heart and learn more compassionate, gentler ways to communicate with their loved ones and other family members.

Module Thirteen: Spiritual Approaches to Coping with Stress

In this training module, participants explore how stress is an inevitable part of the caregiving experience and how best to cope with this stress using spiritual resources. Through stories and exercises they will have the opportunity to practice some spiritual ways of coping with the stress of caregiving.

Module Fourteen: Helping Your Family Member Finish Well

This training module helps family caregivers learn the importance of finding ways to cope with the impending loss of a loved one and of preparing to say goodbye. It explores these issues:

* Recognizing the signs of when it might be time to let go of a loved one

* Understanding the stages of grieving

* Learning how to *be* with a loved one at the end of life

* Learning how to say goodbye

* Understanding hospice care and how it can be helpful

Identifying the spiritual sides to caregiving can help family members find new ways to connect to their loved ones. The caregiving experience can be challenging at times, and spiritual approaches to caring can provide family caregivers with additional support to help them cope and connect in postitive ways.

REFERENCES

Apple Health Care, Inc. *The Better Life Philosophy of Care.* See website: http://www.applehealthcare.com/new/life.shtml.

Bell, V., & Troxel, D. (2001). *The best friends staff: Building a culture of care in Alzheimer's programs.* Baltimore: Health Professions Press.

Fazio, S., Seman, D., & Stansell, J. (1999). *Rethinking Alzheimer's care.* Baltimore: Health Professions Press.

Wellspring Innovative Solutions, Inc. See website: http://www.wellspringis.org.

What Is The Caring Spirit™ Approach?

The Caring Spirit™ is taught in a training program designed to introduce those who work in the field of eldercare and those who are family caregivers to a unique perspective on changing the *culture of caring* in long-term care. *The Caring Spirit* challenges professionals to rethink not only the very definition of caring but how caring is approached and what is involved in providing a caring environment in which professionals and elders can work and live. This program also offers family caregivers new ways to approach caring for their loved ones while also helping them recognize the importance of taking care of themselves.

The Caring Spirit program fills an important gap in existing training: It addresses the *spiritual side* of caring. By infusing spiritual ethics and values into their caregiving efforts, professionals gain an opportunity to experience themselves and their work in positive ways. Care staff can begin to recognize the connection between spirituality and caring. Families, too, learn to recognize the importance of embracing spiritual concepts when caring for their loved ones and themselves. Guiding professionals and families to focus on their own spirits and the spirits of the elders helps to define their work and caring differently.

The Caring Spirit...
- Encourages a compassionate atmosphere that supports the mutuality of caring.
- Supports diversity among professionals and the cultural values of elders.
- Encourages respect for one another in the caring process.
- Recognizes that only cooperation and collaboration can lead to change.
- Helps families recognize how the spirit is involved in caring.
- Helps direct-care workers appreciate the importance of an ethical approach to care that takes into consideration both their own spirits and the spirits of the elders in their care.
- Provides administrators, supervisors, and family members with insight into how to help staff members who are caring for elders feel valued and appreciated for the difficult, and even dangerous, work they do.

The Caring Spirit approach offers solutions and a model of caring that paves the way to approaching care with a new understanding and perspective. The *Caring Spirit* training program presents essential tools for changing how care is provided to elders in this country.

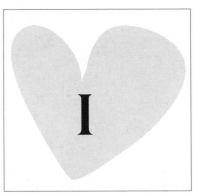

Training for Professional Caregivers

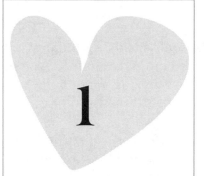

1 Understanding Spirituality and Your Spiritual Self

"There is more to life than merely increasing its speed."
—Mahatma Gandhi

OBJECTIVES

- To help leadership and staff understand the difference between a spiritual model of care and a more traditional model of care

- To define spirituality in its broadest sense and to recognize how diversity is important in providing good spiritual care

- To understand why integrating a spiritual model of care can help staff members see the value in the work they do

- To understand how best to implement a spiritual focus during staff training

A DEFINITION OF SPIRITUALITY

The Caring Spirit training program is unique because the philosophy is based on integrating spiritual values into the training of professional staff in long-term care. By infusing spiritual values, leadership and staff are challenged with providing a more ethical approach to care. In addition, it provides a way for leadership and staff to recognize and understand the importance of their work for fostering greater connection and appreciation.

    The Caring Spirit philosophy defines spirituality broadly as: a way of living in the world in a trusting, peaceful, faithful, and compassionate state; being more aware and conscious of one's surroundings. For some individuals, spirituality is a path for connecting to a higher spirit, thus adhering to a more religious focus. For others, it is a way of connecting to themselves and recognizing something holy either through nature or in other sacred and special ways. For still others, it is both a religious and personal connection.

Spirituality helps us to get in touch with the essence of who we are and how we would like to be in the world. It creates a pathway for us to find meaning and purpose; to make sense of life; and to frame our past, present, and future. When one feels spiritual, one can feel uplifted and honored, respected and valued, cared about and loved.

The Caring Spirit philosophy emphasizes the importance of weaving spiritual values into how staff members care for elders. The most effective way to train those who care for elders is to help these professionals get in touch with their own spiritual side and the spiritual side of elders for whom they care. Helping staff members recognize their own spirituality can result in more meaningful care for our elders—the essential goal of *The Caring Spirit* method.

Family backgrounds, belief systems, cultural expectations, and willingness to be exposed to various spiritual paths all affect the experience of spirituality. There is a delicate balance in helping leadership and staff understand that how they experience spirituality may be quite different from how others experience spirituality, for a variety of reasons. *The Caring Spirit's* training modules guide participants to raise these differences and thus learn about how their different cultural backgrounds affect the way they approach spirituality.

It is my hope that all those who care for elders will develop an increased sensitivity to diversity and expand their definition of spirituality beyond the religious context. Along with introducing the concept of helping staff members draw on their own spiritual resources to provide better care for elders, it is important for staff to understand how spirituality directly affects the lives of elders.

ELDERS AND SPIRITUALITY

For many elders, spirituality encompasses an important part of themselves. As a writer anonymously wrote, "Growing old is one of the ways the soul nudges itself into attention to the spiritual aspect of life. The body's changes teach us about fate, time, nature, mortality, and character. Aging forces us to decide what is important in life."

Studies suggest that as people age, they tend to be drawn to a sense of spirituality and religion, both of which can help them cope with the stresses of aging, provide them with a sense of hope, and enable them to adapt to challenging situations (Crowther, Parker, Achenbaum, Larimore, & Koenig, 2002; Isaia, Parker, & Murrow, 1999; Toughy, 2001). All elders can benefit from activities that nurture their spiritual side. Although few studies to date have explored how spirituality affects elders with dementia, researchers are beginning to consider this area. Fazio, Seman, and Stansell (1999), in *Rethinking Alzheimer's Care,* stated that elders with dementia are able to hold on to the memories of prayers, songs, and rituals that they learned early in life.

Elders with dementia who exhibit behaviors such as wandering, pacing, hoarding, and interrupting often can find solace and a calming of those behaviors when engaged in singing hymns or other religious songs or reading a particular passage from the Bible or other religious documents. Exposure to nature is another spiritual activity that can help to redirect undesirable behavior. Pointing out birds or butterflies in a garden or encouraging elders to look at and smell pretty flowers can help relieve some of the agitated or wandering behavior they can experience with dementia.

When working with elders with dementia, leadership and staff members have witnessed that as the elders' cognitive abilities decline, their ability to relate from the heart becomes more prevalent. They are less interested in facts and more drawn to activities of the heart such as music, crafts, nature, and religion.

When working with elders who are cognitively intact, encouraging their spiritual sides can help them find meaning in the roles and circumstances of later life. Because elders experience more accumulated losses, it is easy for them to feel lonely and isolated. As many elders have shared, they can often feel devalued and detached from the fast-paced world around them. Offering them the opportunity to connect spiritually creates a way to still be in the world. As Ram Dass (2000) so succinctly stated in his book, *Still Here*, "Old age offers the opportunity to shift our cares away from the physical toward what cannot be taken away: our wisdom and the love we offer to those around us." Helping elders connect to themselves and those around them in more spiritual ways can help them feel more connected to life.

Elders who might be experiencing depression or loneliness can often find solace and meaning in being a part of a spirituality group. It seems that listening to spiritual music, for example, helps them access memories that are very soothing and calming. They love reciting prayers that they grew up with or certain passages from sacred texts. Encouraging staff to draw out these memories is important in helping elders in nursing facilities to feel more comfortable and "at home," which can reduce feelings of depression.

THE CARING SPIRIT MODEL OF CARING FOR ELDERS

The traditional medical model's philosophy of care still prevails in many long-term care environments. This model seems to support a more task-oriented, less personal approach to care. *The Caring Spirit* philosophy supports a spiritual model of care as the most successful way to improve the quality of care and life of elders. After learning about *The Caring Spirit* model of care, professionals will be able to see the differences between the two approaches and will embrace a spiritual model of care in their facilities and communities (see Table 1.1).

The spiritual model of care encourages successful training outcomes because it supports a *mutual* experience of understanding and meaning for both the pro-

Table 1.1.   Characteristics of the medical model versus the spiritual model of caring for elders

Medical model	Spiritual model
Staff knows the elder by his or her diagnosis.	Staff recognizes the elder by his or her spirit and soul.
Staff cares for illnesses.	Staff cares for people.
Staff hurries the elder through his or her day.	Staff takes time with the elder.
Staff keeps the elders busy.	Staff provides meaningful activities that nurture the elders' and staff members' spirits.
Staff makes decisions for the elder.	Staff gives choices when appropriate.
Staff treats the elder as a non-person.	Staff treats the elder with dignity and respect.
Elders adapt to the environment.	The environment provides for the spiritual needs of the elders.

fessional providing the care and the care receiver. Spirituality provides the grounding for that mutual experience.

The Caring Spirit philosophy takes caring to a higher level. It allows family members and those who work with elders to recognize that caring for elders is a blessed and sacred act. Caring becomes more than *doing the task,* it becomes *being with* and *caring about* the person.

Using *The Caring Spirit* philosophy, professionals are encouraged to care for elders by embracing the following spiritual values

- Valuing the moment

- Connecting to and from the heart

- Valuing each person as a person and not as a disease

- Valuing spirit and soul

- Maintaining integrity

- Seeing the blessings in the care they are providing

- Having patience

- Valuing the mutuality of caring

- Using humor

- Treasuring each person's essence

- Feeling inspired

- Being respectful of and honoring the person's cultural background and upbringing

Because spirituality knows no racial, economic, ethnic, religious, cultural, age, or gender boundaries, it provides opportunities for staff members and elders to connect in unique and meaningful ways. When we get in touch with our spiritual side, the way of caring for an elder is transformed. We begin to work from the depths of our souls. We act from our hearts. A certain ethical bond is cemented.

In Module 1, which follows, the training emphasis is on helping staff to understand the value of a spiritual approach to care.

REFERENCES

Crowther, M.R., Parker, M.W., Achenbaum, W.A., Larimore, W.L., & Koenig, H.G. (2002). Rowe and Kahn's model of successful aging revisited: Positive spirituality—the forgotten factor. *Gerontologist, 42*(5), 613–620.

Dass, R. (2000). *Still here: Embracing aging, changing, and dying* (p. 24). New York: Riverhead Press.

Fazio, S., Seman, D., & Stansell, J. (1999) *Rethinking Alzheimer's care* (p. 58). Baltimore: Health Professions Press.

Isaia, D., Parker, V., & Murrow, E. (1999). Spiritual well-being among older adults. *Journal of Gerontological Nursing, 25*(8), 15–21.

Touhy, T.A. (2001). Nurturing hope and spirituality in the nursing home. *Holistic Nursing Practice, 15*(4), 45–56.

<table>
<tr><td>♥ | MODULE 1</td><td></td></tr>
</table>

| ♥ MODULE 1 | # Understanding Spirituality and Your Spiritual Self |

"There are only two ways to live your life,
one is as though nothing is a miracle,
the other is as though everything is a miracle."
—Albert Einstein

"What the caterpillar calls the end of of the world,
the master calls a butterfly."
—Richard S. Bach, from *Illusions*

A week prior to the session, the trainer should get word to the participants that they are to bring music that makes them feel spiritual to the first training session.

INTRODUCTION (10 minutes)

Tools Needed
- Flip chart
- Markers

Have each participant introduce him- or herself. If the participant is a staff member, ask him or her to state his or her position. Ask the staff member how long he or she has worked with elders.

Explain to participants what they should expect to learn from this module and list these expectations on the flip chart.
- Participants will have an understanding of spirituality.
- Participants will be more aware of what makes them feel spiritual.
- Participants will be more aware of what makes their co-workers feel spiritual.
- Participants will explore ways to be more spiritual in their work or at home.

Inquire whether participants have other expectations they would like to include; write their expectations on the flip chart.

20

WARM-UP EXERCISE (40 minutes)
Listening to Spiritual Music

> **Tools needed**
> - CD or tape player with good speakers
> - Flip chart
> - Markers

 Question participants about why they were asked to bring in music that made them feel spiritual.

 Spirituality can mean different things to different people. Spirituality
- Is a way to express one's innermost feelings and emotions
- Can open doors to one's self and to one's heart
- Is a way to connect with one's past
- Is a way to connect to others in a deeper manner
- Can provide one with a better understanding of another and help him or her to view another with a new "set of eyes"
- Helps one to learn how to *be* instead of *being busy*

 Have participants listen carefully to each piece of music that is presented. (Play each piece for a minute or two so that participants can get a sense of the piece.)

Have participants think about the following:
- How the music made them feel.
- Why they think their co-worker felt it was spiritual.
- What new information they learned about their co-worker in listening to this piece.

Ask the person presenting the piece how or why the piece made him or her feel spiritual.

Core Exercise (25 minutes)
Defining Spirituality

> **Tools Needed**
> - Flip chart
> - Markers
> - Handout 1.1

Note: The trainer should distribute Handout 1.1, which explains the difference between a medical model and a spiritual model of care.

Have participants help define spirituality. Encourage them to think about words and values that come from being spiritual. Some of the words they might choose include compassion, love, trust, honesty, integrity, loving kindness, faith, spirit, soul, respect, sacred, openness, heart, joy, blessing, healing, God or Lord, higher power or source, human kindness, truth, innermost feelings, prayer, peace, holy, patience, balance, uplifted, honored.

After the participants have given their examples, say "Being spiritual is a way to get in touch with yourself and to connect to others from the heart and soul. It is a way of *being,* not *doing,* in a more aware and conscious state. For some, spirituality becomes a path for connecting to higher power or spirit. For others, it is a way of connecting to the world in a sacred and special way, revealing the holy. It can help you find meaning or purpose, make sense of life, and frame your past. When you feel spiritual, you can feel uplifted, honored, respected, cared for, valued, and loved."

Ask participants what they think about that definition. What would they like to add? Write their comments on the flip chart. Question participants about how they find ways to be "spiritual" in their personal lives? Some ways they might report being spiritual include reading, taking part in sports activities, taking walks on the beach or in the woods, singing, praying, cooking and enjoying nurturing foods, watching a good movie, making love, dancing, connecting with friends and family, playing an instrument, listening to music, meditating, gardening, connecting with nature, enjoying quiet time, and going to church or synagogue.

Ask participants how they might be more "spiritual" in the way they care for elders. Some possible ideas and thoughts include:

- They could share some of their own spiritual ways of being (i.e., taking the residents on a nature walk).
- They could read stories or poetry to elders.
- They could sing to elders.
- They could cook "nourishing" foods with elders.
- They could watch joyful movies with elders.
- They could listen to gospels or other inspirational spiritual music, always making sure that they are sensitive to the elder's religion and cultural heritage.
- They could display some of the characteristics that are more spiritual, such as being loving, patient, caring, joyful, compassionate, and respectful.
- They could stay connected to their own spirits and souls, reaching deep

into their hearts and remembering how they want to be treated and cared about.

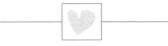

Closing (15 minutes)

Tools Needed
• Handout 1.2

explain   Read to participants the two quotes at the beginning of Module 1.

"There are only two ways to live your life, one is as though nothing is a miracle, the other is as though everything is a miracle."
—Albert Einstein

"What the caterpillar calls the end of life, the master calls a butterfly."
—Richard S. Bach

ask   Question participants about what they think is meant by these quotes in relation to spirituality.

explain   After the participants share their thoughts, share the following about each of the quotes, "The first quote might be about how hope and faith can be available to us, especially if we are willing to open ourselves to those possibilities. It could offer a way of thinking differently when situations in our lives become tough and we feel stuck. It introduces the idea that maybe a miracle could happen. Or the quote could imply that the more positive we are, more positive things might come our way, even under adversity.

"The second quote could serve as a reminder that old age can be just as beautiful as the beginning of life, despite western culture's belief to the contrary. Another interpretation could be that old age can be seen as a time of coming into your own, and beauty can be seen and experienced in different ways as we mature and age."

Distribute Handout 1.2 to participants and read aloud the directions at the top of the page. Encourage participants to try the exercise before the next training session.

ask   Have participants fill out the evaluation form.

Evaluation Questions

1. Did you find this training helpful? (circle one)   Yes   No
   Please explain why or why not.

   _____
   _____
   _____
   _____
   _____

2. How would you define spirituality from *The Caring Spirit* perspective?

   _____
   _____
   _____
   _____

3. Do you believe this information will help you
   to understand how to work more spiritually   Yes   No
   with the elders in your care? (circle one)

   _____
   _____
   _____
   _____

4. Why is it important to bring your spirit to work?

   _____
   _____
   _____
   _____

5. How did you feel after this workshop? (circle all that apply)

good	encouraged	cared about
sad	bored	listened to
frustrated	informed	angry
blessed	joyful	inspired
motivated	good about myself	

Medical Versus Spiritual Model of Care

Medical model	Spiritual model
Staff knows the elder by his or her diagnosis.	Staff recognizes the elder by his or her spirit and soul.
Staff cares for illnesses.	Staff cares for people.
Staff hurries the elder through his or her day.	Staff takes time with the elder.
Staff keeps the elder busy.	Staff provides meaningful activities that nurture each elder's and staff person's spirits.
Staff makes decisions for the elder.	Staff gives choices when appropriate.
Staff treats the elder as a non-person.	Staff treats the elder with dignity and respect.
Elders adapt to the environment.	The environment provides for the spiritual needs of the elders.

Faith, Life, Love

This handout is to help you find ways to connect to the spiritual sides of yourselves. The main objective of this exercise is to help you find a way to bring spirituality more into your lives. Each letter stands for a spiritual concept. It is suggested that each day, you pick a letter from the Faith, Life, or Love column. After picking the letter, you can reflect on what that letter represents and how you can incorporate the concept throughout the day. For example, if you pick from the Faith column, letter F, decide who in your life you may need to forgive. Or if you pick letter I in the Faith column, think about how to "keep the faith" when you feel that things are challenging or stressful.

FAITH

F—Forgive and forget transgressions for whatever reason.
A—Accept people for who they are and try not to judge.
I—Involve yourself in prayer and keep the faith.
T—Teach yourself to be patient and tolerant.
H—Help others who are not able to help themselves.

LIFE

L—Live each moment as if it could be your last.
I—Invite others into your life, even those you might not think to invite.
F—Find yourself a friend you can trust.
E—Empty your heart and mind each night before you go to sleep.

LOVE

L—Lend a hand to those in need.
O—Open your heart and listen.
V—Vent your feelings honestly and lovingly.
E—Engage in life and believe in yourself.

Creating a Spiritual Work Environment

2

"At the very least, if leaders provide a clear sense of direction
and provide feedback along the way, they encourage people
to reach inside and do their best. Encouraging the heart
accomplishes something else essential to excellence…
It speaks to people's hearts—to deeply held values
and beliefs, to something beyond the material—and
contributes to creating meaning in the workplace."
—James Kouzes & Barry Posner, from *Encouraging the Heart*

OBJECTIVES

- To define what is meant by a *Caring Spirit* work environment

- To help leadership understand how the environment in which staff members work affects their morale, job satisfaction, and performance

- To identify ways that leadership can influence the staff's work environment to create a sense of positive spirit

EFFECT OF THE ENVIRONMENT ON THE SPIRIT OF THE STAFF

Experts in the field of long-term care have begun to examine the importance of creating a different kind of nursing care environment. Examples of ways that leaders in the field are creating new environments can be found in the work of the following authors:

- In their book *The Best Friends Staff,* Bell and Troxel stress the importance of

27

encouraging friendlier interaction between residents and staff members.

- In *The Eden Alternative,* author William H. Thomas believes that environments need to feel welcoming, homey, and meaningful for residents.

- In *Rethinking Alzheimer's Care,* authors Fazio, Seman, and Stansell encourage more connection among staff, families, and elders and the *rethinking* of what caring environments should look like.

The physical and emotional environment in which we work influences how we feel about our jobs. The environment reflects "the spirit and caring" of the staff members and elders who work and live within it. When the building is clean, has a warm and homelike feeling, smells good, and when the staff and leadership are caring and warm toward the elders, it sends the message that this is a community with leadership that cares—this is a caring community. There is a sense of ownership and pride among the staff members and elders who work and live within such an environment. When an environment is not warm, welcoming, and well run, it often appears that there is little sense of ownership and pride.

Over the years, I have asked staff members who work in long-term care what type of environment they would like to work in, and they have shared the following reflections:

"I would like my environment to smell better and feel good."

"I would like the physical environment to have a lot of windows and be brightly lit and painted."

"I would enjoy an environment that made me feel more at home."

"I want my work environment to reflect my interests and values."

"The most enjoyable environment would be one where we were all like friends."

"I would enjoy having more time to be with the residents and my co-workers to get to know them better."

"I would like a warm, caring environment where my supervisors showed me they cared."

"I would like a warm, caring environment where fun was encouraged with my co-workers and the residents."

The message in their responses is simple: Leadership must create environments that foster a sense of belonging, encourage relationships, feel homey, are clean, and feel alive. Leadership must create environments in which staff can feel at home.

HOW TO ENCOURAGE A *CARING SPIRIT* WORK ENVIRONMENT

A *Caring Spirit* work environment is physically comfortable, provides space for staff members to replenish themselves, feels good to work in, encourages ways for staff members to know one another, and makes the staff feel that the leadership cares. It supports a spiritual approach to care. It encourages staff members to draw on their personal spiritual resources to help them through their day and creates a sense of spirit in the environment that is joyful, uplifting, calming, warm, comfortable, safe, and caring.

To create a *Caring Spirit* work environment, leadership must be committed to providing the necessary time and resources. The staff in long-term care has a very challenging job. In most facilities, each staff member is responsible for taking care of 8–10 residents per shift. In addition, many of the residents they care for are either emotionally or physically challenging because of their illnesses and life situations. The staff is charged with providing quality and compassionate care, although it is difficult to imagine how these caregivers can to do so in the type of environments in which they so often work. It is essential for the leadership to recognize these hardships and provide staff members with the needed support and supervision. In addition, the leadership must rethink and commit to the four basics needed to create a *Caring Spirit* environment. A discussion of each follows.

THE FOUR BASICS: HOW TO CREATE A *CARING SPIRIT* IN THE WORK ENVIRONMENT

1. **Leadership must be willing to spend time in the environment in which the staff works.**

Why do so many department heads and leaders of residential care facilities have offices separate from where the staff works and the elders live? Management research strongly supports the importance of leadership that is visible to staff members and families (Kouzes & Posner, 1999). Being visible demonstrates to staff and families that leadership cares and is aware of what is happening in the environment. "Hanging out" in the staff's work environment has a lot of value, according to the authors of the book *Encouraging the Heart.* Families consistently share one fear—that the leadership is not around to supervise and motivate the staff and to keep an observant eye on the environment in which their loved ones live. They worry about how the lack of consistent leadership affects the care of their family members. I initially had similar concerns when placing my mother in an assisted living facility and then in the nursing home where she currently lives. When I had confidence that the community's leadership was supervising and staying involved with the staff, I felt more comfortable and peaceful about her placement.

2. **Leadership must recognize the effect of the environment on the staff.**

How can any leadership believe that staff members could be happy or motivated to work in environments that are physically unappealing, unsafe, cold, and unwelcoming? Would they be motivated to work in a depressing environment? When an environment is clean, safe, attractive, warm, welcoming, and smells good, it reflects the values of the leadership. When staff members feel good about where they work and for whom they work, the overall care they provide is better.

3.   Leadership must be willing to encourage relationships.

Managerial myth says that leaders must not establish relationships with their workers. However, extensive research supports the importance of relationships in the work environment. Paraphrasing the authors of *Encouraging the Heart*, people will work more effectively and harder for people they like (Kouzes & Posner, 1999). If leadership is willing to encourage relationships, the overall environment will be a more pleasant place to work and live. Retention is much higher in the environments in which

- Staff members have relationships with one another.

- The facility leadership provides informal gatherings for staff members.

- The leadership emphasizes the importance of providing time for staff members to get to know one another.

4.   Leadership must be willing to create a culture of celebration and recognition.

In the book *Corporate Celebration: Play, Purpose, and Profit at Work*, authors Deal and Key share the following: "Celebration provides the symbolic adhesive that welds a community together." They further state, "Celebrations infuse life with passion and purpose... They bond people together and connect us to shared values and myths" (Kouzes & Posner, 1999). Staff feel more positive and motivated to remain in their jobs and perform well in environments in which they are celebrated. The work done by The Center for Creative Leadership and other management research supports this observation as well (Campbell, 1984; Kouzes & Posner, 1995).

HONORING STAFF

The William Breman Jewish Home (WBJH) in Atlanta, Georgia, is a wonderful example of a long-term care environment that recognizes the importance of relationships and of honoring the staff. The WBJH always has made it a priority to honor and celebrate its staff with recognition of families' births and deaths and holidays that are meaningful to the staff members such as Martin Luther King Day and Kwanzaa.

I will never forget the going-away party that staff members created for their Executive Director, affectionately known as Deb. She had been their director for more than 20 years and was moving back to her hometown in New Jersey. Each department participated in heartwarming skits and songs about Deb—some funny and some very sentimental. The dietary department went out of its way to provide the special foods Deb loved. The activities department decorated the room and each table with mementos that were meaningful to Deb. When the rather shy, big, burly men on the maintenance staff performed a song and skit they had written for her, I was amazed and touched. Even staff members who had retired came back to participate and to say goodbye. Demonstrating her role as a leader who values relationships, Deb had set aside a part of the room for staff members to have their picture taken with her and with one another. She wanted to make sure she marked the event and their relationship! As I watched how the staff honored and respected Deb and how she did the same, I had tears in my eyes. I thought, "This is a community that exemplifies *The Caring Spirit.*"

Training Module 2, Creating a Spiritual Work Environment, will help inspire and motivate professionals to create environments like the WBJH has.

REFERENCES

Bell, V., & Troxel, D. (2001). *The Best Friends staff: Building a culture of care in Alzheimer's programs.* Baltimore: Health Professions Press.

Campbell, D. (1984). *If I'm in charge here, why is everybody laughing?* Greensboro, NC: Center for Creative Leadership.

Fazio, S., Seman, D., & Stansell, J. (1999). *Rethinking Alzheimer's care.* Baltimore: Health Professions Press.

Kouzes, J.M., & Posner, B.Z. (1995). *The leadership challenge: How to keep getting extraordinary things done in organizations* (2nd ed.). San Francisco: Jossey-Bass Press.

Kouzes, J.M., & Posner, B.Z. (1999). *Encouraging the heart: A leader's guide to rewarding and recognizing others.* San Francisco: Jossey-Bass Press.

Thomas, W.H. (1996). *Life worth living: How someone you love can still enjoy life in a nursing home—The Eden Alternative in action.* Acton, MA: VanderWyk & Burnham.

<table>
<tr><td>

♥   **MODULE 2**

</td><td>

Creating a Spiritual Work Environment

</td></tr>
</table>

> "It is the human environment, not the
> physical environment, that frequently has the
> greatest influence on the culture of a place and
> how people act and function in a particular setting."
> —Fazio, Seman, & Stansell, from *Rethinking Alzheimer's Care*

INTRODUCTION (15 minutes)

Tools Needed
• Flip chart
• Markers

 Have participants introduce themselves, and ask them what they think is meant by "creating a spiritual work environment"?

 Explain to participants what they should expect to learn from this module and list these objectives on the flip chart.
- Participants will have a clearer understanding of what a spiritual environment looks and feels like.
- Participants will explore together ideas to help create a more spiritual environment.
- Participants will examine how each staff member can find ways to infuse spirituality into the workplace.

 Ask participants if there are other expectations they would like to include, and write those on the flip chart.

WARM-UP EXERCISE (30 minutes)
Defining Home

Tools Needed
- Flip chart
- Markers
- Paper and pens
- Handout 2.1

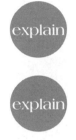

explain Tell participants that one of the essential ingredients for creating a spiritual work environment is finding ways for staff and elders to feel *at home* in their environment.

explain Tell participants that mental health professionals define the meaning of *home* as a place
- In which they can feel safe and secure
- In which they are loved and cared for
- In which they have privacy and experience intimacy
- In which they feel comfortable not only in the external environment but also *internally*
- In which they are free to be themselves
- That provides a "container" for relationships, personal things, and for their own selves
- In which they feel a sense of belonging

ask Have participants divide into groups of two or three. Ask participants to think about how they would define home using Handout 2.1. Have one person record participants' comments.

ask Have participants share with the group how they answered the questions. Write some of their comments on the flip chart.

explain Explain to participants that although there are positive definitions of home (e.g., the ones described above), for some people home may not be such a positive experience. There are people who come from broken homes or homes with abuse or neglect. Thus, it is important to be aware and sensitive to these situations for staff members and elders.

Core Exercise (40 minutes)
Creating a Spiritual Workplace

"The world we see is the world we carry with us."
—Anonymous

> **Tools Needed**
> - CD or tape player
> - Flip chart
> - Markers

Have participants share what they think the above quote means and write their responses on the flip chart. You might want to share the following:
- The "world" we see is very individual and affects us personally.
- How we view our environment will affect how we think about it and behave in response to it.
- What we see affects how we feel.
- How we see things affects our perspective toward much of what we experience.

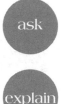

Ask participants to think about ways in which they can create a more spiritual work environment for themselves. Write responses on the flip chart.

Provide participants with some additional ideas, such as
- Listening to music that helps them to feel spiritual during their break time. Staff members have shared that just listening to music cleanses their souls and makes it easier to go back to work.
- Singing while working. I will always remember a caregiver who sang while he took care of his residents; not only did they love it, but it made him feel good too!
- Bringing in snack foods that are nourishing to the soul, such as fruit, vegetables, cheese, and other foods that are more apt to help them feel energized and feel good. Staff members could ask management to provide some of these foods for them as well.
- Getting outside on nice days, even just to breathe the fresh air or take a brief walk.
- Creating a space in the environment that is specifically decorated to soothe their souls and replenish their spirit. I recall one inpatient hospice in which staff members took over a small room that they painted a soothing color, furnished comfortably, and outfitted with nice-smelling incense and soft music.
- Thinking of their jobs in more spiritual ways, for example housekeepers are "keepers of the house," caregivers are "angels" or "ministers of

service," food service workers are "people who feed elders' souls and spirits," maintenance workers are "healers of the physical house."

 Have participants share one reason why they think it is important to create a more spiritual work environment. How will it affect the way they feel about their work, themselves, and the elders for whom they care? Write their responses on the flip chart.

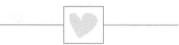

Closing (5 minutes)
Summarize

 Mention that you hope that participants will begin to work toward creating a more *spiritual, homelike environment* in their workplace.

 Have participants fill out the evaluation form.

Evaluation Questions

1. Did you find this training helpful? (circle one)   Yes   No
   Please explain why or why not.

   _____
   _____
   _____
   _____

2. What are some ways you could create a more spiritual environment at work?

   _____
   _____
   _____
   _____

3. How might creating a more spiritual environment impact your morale?
   List at least two examples.

   _____
   _____
   _____
   _____

4. How did you feel after this workshop? (circle all that apply)

good	encouraged	cared about
sad	bored	listened to
frustrated	informed	angry
blessed	joyful	inspired
motivated	good about myself	

Questions to Ponder: Defining Home

"The world we see is the world we carry with us."
—Anonymous

- What does home mean to you?

- What are some characteristics of home?

- When do you feel most "at home"?

- Can you feel "at home" even if you do not have a home?

- How could work feel more like home?

- What is meant by "home is where the heart is"?

Why Working in Eldercare Is a Blessing

3

OBJECTIVES

- To highlight the importance of helping staff members see how their work provides them with *blessings*

- To reveal for care staff and leadership the blessings of working in long-term care

- To define the term *conscious caring*

WHAT BLESSING MEANS IN THE WORKPLACE

Like spirituality, the word *blessing* can hold many different meanings for people. The Merriam-Webster Dictionary alone has seven entries under *blessing*, one of which holds particular meaning for *The Caring Spirit* program. This definition is "to invoke divine care for."

Invoking divine care is a blessing that the staff can provide when caring for elders. Framing the effect of their care of elders as a blessing can be very powerful to staff members, as evidenced by the following comments from staff members after participating in Module 3 of *The Caring Spirit* training.

> "Seeing elders as blessings reminds us that we are inspirations to our residents."

> "I am able to see just how important what we do is and be proud of what I am doing."

> "I feel moved, touched, and enlightened that they feel that I care about them and respect their feelings."

> "I realize about myself that I need to be thankful for my life and the people around."

CONSCIOUS CARING: OUR WORK IS A BLESSING

The Caring Spirit training program attempts to provide a different perspective on caring for elders. Helping staff members to understand the blessings of their work and how blessing those they care for and work with promotes a positive sense of spirit is paramount to ensuring the total health of elders and the staff who work with them.

Caring for elders should be seen as a sacred act. Our culture, however, tends to view this work as a burden. Teaching staff about blessings and the role they play is a powerful way to begin to change culture.

In the book *The Path of Blessing*, Rabbi Marcia Prager (2003) shared some interesting thoughts about blessing. She stated that "blessing implies a transfer of intention, hopefulness… If I bless you, I seek to move something of myself toward you, I want you to feel richer, more hopeful. I am offering you something by blessing you."

Thinking about the blessings of caring in this way has inspired me to consider how we can care for elders in a completely different way—a term I call *conscious caring*. I define *conscious caring* as caring for elders in an intentional, sensitive, compassionate, respectful, and loving way. The key word is intentional. Implicit in this approach to care is the belief that the way you care for someone affects the experience between you and the elder for whom you care. It implies, "I am blessing you through my caring for you, and you are blessing me by allowing me to do so." It also means taking caring beyond the mere performance of the task by caring about the process of how the task is accomplished. Conscious caring brings forth a sense of pride in one's daily tasks. It takes caring to an intimate level by associating caring with blessing. Working with elders affords professionals the opportunity to apply conscious caring to their work every day. Reminding professionals and caregivers of the blessings they give and receive can help them feel more appreciative of their work and creates positive morale and job satisfaction.

I continually appreciate how blessed I am to have the opportunity to help elders finish well. I feel blessed to be in the presence of these resilient, wise people. There is not a day that goes by that I do not learn something from them. My life has been shaped by their attitudes about life; no matter how difficult their lives have been, they find a way to see the blessings in their lives. Recognizing the events, people, or gifts in life as blessings helps one feel the presence of something divine.

Author John Morton, in his book *The Blessings Already Are,* supports the importance of blessings in people's lives. He takes the conscious concept one step further by encouraging people to see that "the blessings already are." He believes that not only is it important to recognize the blessings that are possible but also to recognize the blessings we already have in our lives. He stated, "Sometimes the most meaningful aspects of life are often ones that seem ordinary and inconsequential. We often miss or take for granted the many blessings in our lives, overlooking them as just part of everyday life" (Morton, 2000).

Dr. Rachel Naomi Remen supports Morton's philosophy. She points out in her book, *My Grandfather's Blessings,* how the simple, ordinary things that we do can affect those around us in profound ways. She cites the following examples:

- The difference it can make for someone when one says something kind

- When one touches someone by hugging or holding one's hand

- The willingness to listen quietly and generously

- A warm smile or wink of recognition

"Everything in the world needs blessings. If the holy or higher power has made all things, it is up to us to strengthen them, feed them, and free them. The capacity to bless life is in everybody. Blessing life moves us closer to each other and closer to our authentic selves" (Remen, 2000).

VALIDATING THE WORK OF STAFF

When training staff members in long-term care, it is important to focus some sessions solely on validating the difficult work they do. Although our culture does not seem to value this work, we, as professionals, must. Professionals need to help care staff recognize the things that seem to be ordinary tasks in daily work, but are actually examples of blessing life. Rabbi Prager, in her book *The Path of Blessing,* offers an interesting perspective that begins to address this point. She illustrates a beautiful example by sharing how effortlessly children see the blessings in the world. As she states, "When we look at small children, we see their sense of wonder, their openness to the miraculous. When we allow the daily miracles to be passed by, our openness to the abundance of divine blessing withers" (Prager, 2003).

It seems that as we grow into adulthood, we lose our curiosity, our delight in the simple things, and our willingness to stay open to the many blessings all around us. As we grow more habituated, less connected to one another, and busier, we lose awareness of blessings.

To help staff members develop greater sensitivity to the potential around them and recognize the blessings, I suggest that professionals consider the work of John Morton, who has defined 10 blessings that are always available to us in our lives.

- **Loving:** Morton describes loving as something that comes naturally to people. Everyone needs to feel and be loved and everyone has love within him- or herself. He points out that, "if everyone were entirely loving, nothing would matter." He adds, "when love is present, there is an 'ecstatic' relationship to everything."

- **Caring:** According to Morton, caring is an extension of loving. He states that "caring is how loving makes itself known."

- **Sharing:** Sharing, in turn, is an extension of caring. Only when we share our loving and caring toward one another and the elders with whom we work can caring and loving be possible.

- **Health:** Health is something natural, as it is one way we love who we are. Health reminds us that we are blessed to have our bodies and that our bodies are a home to our souls. Health reminds us how sacred our bodies truly are.

- **Wealth, Abundance, Riches, and Prosperity:** Morton believes that wealth is manifest in abundance, prosperity, and riches. Wealth is seen as the many blessings that are all around and within us. He stresses that wealth is not about the material, but rather about what is emotional and spiritual. When we can recognize the riches we have in our lives through our friends, family, pets, and spiritual beliefs, we can appreciate all of the abundance and the richness in our lives.

- **Happiness:** Happiness is created through ourselves and our interpretations of how we see our lives. It is available to us in the present moment.

- **Touching:** Touching is the way we physically express and experience our blessings; it is how we connect. People need to feel connected at every stage of their lives. To survive and thrive, we need to touch and to be touched.

These 10 blessings are an excellent way to introduce the concept of *conscious caring* and demonstrate how professionals have these blessings available to them every day. Helping staff members think about how to apply these blessings to their work with elders and in their personal lives is the focus of Module 3. Staff will learn the following:

- Why the work they do is truly a blessing

- How to recognize the blessings in their lives

- The many ways they feel blessed to work with each other

- How to bless themselves

REFERENCES

Merriam-Webster collegiate dictionary (10th ed.). (2002). Springfield, MA: Merriam-Webster.

Morton, J. (2000). *The blessings already are.* Los Angeles: Mandeville Press.

Prager, M. (2003). *The path of blessing: Experiencing the energy and abundance of the divine.* Woodstock, VT: Jewish Lights Publishing.

Remen, R.N. (2000). *My grandfather's blessings: Stories of strength, refuge and belonging.* New York: Riverhead Books.

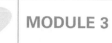

Why Working in Eldercare Is a Blessing

"Anytime we share someone's joy,
we bless the life in them."
—Rachel Naomi Remen, from *My Grandfather's Blessings*

"When your life is full of love, your life is fully blessed.
The task is to always walk the path of loving in all ways."
—John Morton, from *The Blessings Already Are*

INTRODUCTION (20 minutes)

Tools Needed
• Flip chart
• Markers

 Have participants introduce themselves.

 Explain to participants what they should expect to learn from this module and list these expectations on the flip chart.
• Participants will better understand why working with elders is a blessing.
• Participants will have an opportunity to become more aware of the blessings in their lives.
• Participants will be able to experience the many ways they feel blessed to work with each other and to recognize the abundance they receive from their jobs.

 Share with participants the two quotes in the beginning of this module. Ask them to comment on what the quotes mean. Share meanings as well as the concept of *conscious caring*. Summarize for attendees John Morton's belief that 10 blessings are given to us once we are born.

WARM -UP EXERCISE (30 minutes)
We Are Blessed

> Tools Needed
> - White construction paper
> - Markers
> - Clear tape

Tell the participants that this exercise helps them to appreciate the blessings that result from their work.

Each participant is to help another participant tape construction paper onto his or her back. Then each participant is to write on the paper why they feel *blessed* to work with each of their co-workers. They are to write whatever comes from their hearts.

After everyone has written something on each other's backs, ask the participants to remove the construction paper from their backs. Give each participant a few minutes to read and absorb what has been written about him or her.

Ask the participants to share what was written on their papers by answering the questions that follow.
- How do you feel about what was written?
- Does it help you to see your work differently?
- Was there a blessing that surprised you?
- If you were to have picked a blessing for yourself, what would it have been?

CORE EXERCISE (20 minutes)
Making a Difference

Tell the participants that you are going to read them a short story. Ask them to pay attention to how this story is similar to their work lives and maybe even to their personal lives.

Making a Difference (the story)
There was an old man walking along the beach at low tide, picking up starfish drying in the sun and gently throwing them back into the ocean. He has been doing this for some time when a jogger overtakes him and asks what he is doing. The old man explains that the starfish will die in the sun, and so he is throwing them back into the ocean. Astounded, the younger man begins to laugh: "Why, old fellow, don't waste your time. Can't you

see that there are hundreds and hundreds of starfish on this beach? And thousands of beaches in this world? And another low tide tomorrow? What makes you think that you can make a difference?" And still laughing, he runs on down the beach.

The old man looks after him for a long while. Then he walks on and before long he passes another starfish. Stooping, he picks it up and looks at it thoughtfully. Then gently, he throws it back into the ocean. "Made a difference to that one," he says to himself...

...When it comes down to it, no matter how great or how small the need, we can only bless one life at a time. (From *My Grandfather's Blessings,* by Rachel Naomi Remen)

 Ask the participants the following questions:
* Do you feel it was silly of the old man to throw back the starfish?
* How are this old man's actions similar to caring for elders?
* Do you always know when you are making a difference?
* How do you think you are making a difference in the lives of the elders with whom you work?
* How do you make a difference with the people in your own life?

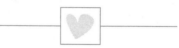

CLOSING (10 minutes)

 Ask participants to share one blessing they received from this training today.

Reinforce that participants are to bring an inspirational poem, saying or quote, or short reading to the next training session.

Have participants fill out the evaluation form.

Evaluation Questions

1. Did you find this training helpful? (circle one)   Yes   No
   Please explain why or why not.

   _____
   _____
   _____
   _____

2. Why is it important to see your work as a *blessing?*

   _____
   _____
   _____
   _____

3. What *blessings* are you now able to see since you attended this workshop?

   _____
   _____
   _____
   _____

4. How did you feel after this workshop? (circle all that apply)

good	encouraged	cared about
sad	bored	listened to
frustrated	informed	angry
blessed	joyful	inspired
motivated	good about myself	

4 How Inspiration Affects Staff Members and Those for Whom They Care

"Really believe in your heart of hearts that your fundamental purpose, the reason for being, is to enlarge the lives of others. Your life will be enlarged also. And all of the other things we have been taught to concentrate on will take care of themselves."
—Peter Thigpen, Executive Reserves

OBJECTIVES

- To help leadership recognize the importance of learning how to inspire the staff who work in long-term care settings

- To suggest ways to encourage inspiration and motivation in the workplace

- To provide ways for leadership to help staff members recognize how they inspire one another and the elders for whom they care and how the elders may inspire them

RECOGNIZING THE EFFECT OF INSPIRATION IN THE WORKPLACE

A major concern in long-term care environments is the lack of inspiration shown by the leaders of facilities toward the staff. How can leaders expect their staff to be motivated and perform at a high level without inspiration? In order to motivate the staff, however, we must first determine what motivates and inspires staff members to perform well.

49

Staff members consistently relate that they feel motivated to perform well when their supervisors

- Recognize the need for encouragement and feeling valued

- Demonstrate through words and actions that they value the staff as workers

- Make a point to involve staff members in decision making as well as asking for their opinions

- Take the time to observe staff members working and then point out what they see as the staff members' strengths, not just their weaknesses

- Model behavior that demonstrates a willingness to help the staff out in crisis times and at other times

- Share with the staff some of the challenges the leaders face in their work and acknowledge who has inspired them to get through those challenges

- Take the time to listen to staff concerns and then work collaboratively with staff members to find solutions

- Take the time to supervise them and to inspire them to do a good job

When reflecting on these responses from the staff, it is clear that these simple but incredibly important suggestions should be in the forefront of every supervisor's mind. They further reinforce the belief that inspiration is a key ingredient in boosting positive staff morale, job satisfaction, and performance.

WHAT THE RESEARCH SAYS

Researchers, who have evaluated the challenges of staff morale, job satisfaction, and performance, have examined many factors that appear to have a great affect. One factor prevalent in all types of work environments, particularly in long-term care facilities, is the importance of being inspired and encouraged to do a good job and then valued and appreciated for doing so (Kouzes & Posner, 1999; Parsons, Parker, Ghose, 1998; Schaefer & Moos, 1996). Considering that staff in long-term care settings are not highly reimbursed for their work, this seems to be a critical factor.

One of the many studies regarding work satisfaction among staff members in nursing homes found that interpersonal relationships were most important for stable staff. Getting along with their co-workers and supervisors was a very important indicator for remaining on the job. In addition, the study found that next in importance was supervision, achievement, and responsibility. Knowing what their supervisors expected of them, being able to accomplish their tasks, and feeling responsible for their work, made staff members feel most satisfied with their jobs (Parsons, Simmons, Penn, & Furlough, 2003)

An alarming study, and one that needs to be carefully considered by long-term care leadership, was conducted by Peter Fitzpatrick (2002), an associate professor of health care management. After extensively examining the research on turnover and job satisfaction in long-term care, he concluded that there should be a heightened sense of urgency on the part of leadership in long-term care to attend to the problems of turnover, job dissatisfaction, and low staff morale. He pointed to two realities:

1. By 2030, 19% of the population will be over the age of 65 (nearly 70 million people) and approximately 5.3 million elders will require nursing home or 24-hour care.

2. There will be an overwhelming need for certified nursing assistants and a shortage of these workers is projected.

This issue will not go away. It needs to be made a priority and given the attention it so deserves. One simple way to begin to address this issue is to recognize staff members for the work they do.

The authors of *Encouraging the Heart* and *The Leadership Challenge* (Kouzes & Posner, 1999 & 1995) reviewed much of the research on job satisfaction and job performance and the effect of leadership on these areas. After evaluating the literature they concluded that staff members are often "starved for recognition." In addition, they found that the leader's ability to inspire people to become the best they can be may be the most critical skill of good leaders! Everyone needs to be encouraged to reach their highest potential and then be reinforced to remain there. Inspiring a staff member to perform to his or her highest potential involves a willingness to invest time, money, and attention. It means caring about the person, recognizing the person's strengths and expertise, and encouraging the person's spirit. Author David Whyte, in his book *The Heart Aroused,* suggested that corporate America needs to rethink what it means to "arouse the heart and soul" of the worker. He contended that soul is the "hidden and neglected side of corporate life."

The 21st century brings forth a significantly different landscape for work and home life than in the past. Work and home life are more complex and stressful, and the landscape is continually changing. The majority of Americans spend 8–14 hours per day in the workplace. To provide balance between work and family life, the workplace will need to provide more support than just a place to work and a paycheck. "Creative leaders find ways of stepping into the shoes of other people and asking, 'How would I feel and what would I want if I were this person?'" (Hendricks and Ludeman, 1997).

ENCOURAGING INSPIRATION

Inspiration is a key factor in developing a positive work culture. Inspiration encourages one to feel motivated, moved, enlivened, connected, energized, and hopeful. Bringing inspiration into workers' lives is critical to reaching the goals of lower turnover and higher job satisfaction and performance.

The following are suggestions for ways that leadership can encourage inspiration in the long-term care workplace:

1. **Leadership must recognize the importance and value of encouraging workers to feel inspired and cared about.**

Finding creative ways to thank and praise staff is essential. Leadership needs to set aside time for the sole purpose of inspiring staff. In one assisted living community where I consulted, I recommended that the leadership create a "Taking Care of Your Spirits Day" for the staff. Volunteers were recruited to provide the following sessions: massages, nail care, pedicures, facials, chiropractic assessments, and hair styling and cutting. Staff members could choose two sessions. They loved the attention and care given to them and felt recognized. This has now become a twice-a-year event!

Training is not only for disseminating information to staff but also for motivating, encouraging, and inspiring staff members to perform at their highest level. Finding training time in long-term care is a very real challenge. With all of the state requirements and liability challenges, it is easy to push aside time for encouraging the heart. If we do not find training time for encouraging and inspiring our staff, however, we will continue the vicious cycle of low staff morale, poor job performance, and high turnover. This not only greatly affects the quality of care for elders, but also takes a toll on the financial bottom line with tremendous turnover expense, risk of liability, and reputation.

2. **Leadership needs to set clear goals for performance.**

We all need to know what is expected of us. If we are involved in a collaborative process, we will take more ownership of the goals we have set forth because we can be held accountable in a very personal way to accomplish them. Management literature supports this attitude and adds the caveat that incentives and rewards are critical in reinforcing follow-through of goals. In one nursing home where I have consulted for more than 10 years, the turnover rate was less than half of the 120% industry standard. This nursing home has consistently found ways to involve staff in decision making and to recognize the need for fostering staff growth and success.

3. **Leadership needs to recognize encouragement as a form of feedback and continuous evaluation.**

Leadership needs to set aside time to provide feedback and observe staff more than once a year. In addition, it is important for leadership to implement creative and meaningful recognition programs.

4. **Leadership has to demonstrate that it believes in the staff members and feels inspired by them!**

A compliment goes a long way, especially if it is given from the heart by a supervisor or mentor. When a leader takes the time to compliment or share how inspired he or she feels by watching that particular worker, the effect can have a lasting effect.

I will never forget one staff member I was working with in an assisted living facility. She was in her sixties and had been a caregiver in long-term care for more than 30 years. Her supervisor told me that this particular caregiver was impatient and not very kind toward the residents she cared for. She was considering letting the worker go. As I watched this caregiver, I could see that she was tired, stressed, and unmotivated. I wondered how she felt about her work all these years. I sat with her and asked her how long she had been working with elders. After she told me, I asked her how she liked her work and asked her how she stayed connected to her heart and spirit after all these years. Her reaction was fascinating. Her face brightened and she said, "You know, I loved this work. I have felt like I am serving these people and that is what God put me on this earth to do. But these past 2 years, I have felt tired and worn out." I asked her how she might get back in touch with her original purpose for doing this work and she then stated, "I need to remind myself why I am doing this work and pray about it." When I saw her interacting later in the day with her residents, I noticed a very different approach. She was kinder, gentler, and more patient. I approached her and said to her, "Well, I guess you must have had a prayer or two answered. How fortunate these residents are to have you as their angel to care for them!" She smiled.

INNOVATIVE INSPIRATIONAL PROGRAMS

The following are some simple activities that I have found to be successful in inspiring workers.

- *"The Compliment Cards" Program.* Compliment cards are small index-size cards that families, supervisors, or other staff members can fill out when they see someone doing a great job. These cards are given to the staff member receiving the compliment and also placed in the employee's file. When a staff person gathers a designated number of these cards, he or she can turn them in for Wal-Mart dollars.

- *"The Caring Jar" Program.* This program involves encouraging family members or volunteers to write complimentary messages about staff. These are collected in a jar then read by management at staff meetings.

- *"Taking Care of Staff Day" Program.* This program was developed so that families could thank staff members for their hard work and kind efforts. Families recruit volunteer professionals to provide a day of R & R for the staff, such as massages, nail care, facials, Tai Chi, and so forth.

- *"Improve Workers' Lives" Programs.* This program looks for ways to help reduce staff stress by 1) establishing an employee-run food cooperative, 2) offering the use of vans for employee carpools, and 3) contracting with a landlord for low-cost housing (Packer-Tursman, 1996).

Most people have known at least one or two individuals who have affected them so deeply and profoundly that it is often hard to describe in words how they felt. When I think about my own life, I know that if I didn't have people to inspire me, I never would have attempted half the things I have accomplished in my life, such as writing this book! People who inspire can affect others' lives in very profound ways. These beacons connect to the very essence of others and gently nudge them toward the things they fear the most and want to accomplish in their lives. People who inspire often connect others to the parts of themselves that may be hidden or that yearn to grow and develop. It is through this inspirational connection that they can reach into the soul of another.

Situations that inspire also can be very powerful and tap into one's heart. For example, think about the numerous tragedies that the Kennedy family has endured over the years and how they were able to continue to maintain strength and courage toward life. They are true inspirations! Another inspirational example is Dr. Martin Luther King, Jr., who had the faith and belief that all people could live together in harmony and draw strength from one another. He had the courage to speak out and to hold fast to his dreams in a society that was judgmental and often unkind. Also consider the Dalai Lama who, despite experiencing the displacement of his people from their country, held onto hope and compassion and pledged his life to the needs of humankind. Ordinary individuals can also inspire, touching one life at a time with their unconditional love and kindness.

Inspirational situations touch people's lives in very profound ways. In order to recognize them, however, people have to take the time to appreciate and draw these situations into their lives.

Module 4 was created out of the strong conviction that many of the staff members who care for elders are not aware of how much of an inspiration they are to elders and their families. In fact, they often serve as an inspiration to all who know them.

This training module helps leadership encourage staff members to appreciate and become more aware of

- Who has inspired them the most in their lives

- What inspiration means to them

- How they might be inspired by working with elders to help them "finish well"

- How they can inspire each other

REFERENCES

Fitzpatrick, P.G. (2002). Turnover of certified nursing assistants: A major problem for long-term care facilities. *Hospital Topics: Research and Perspectives on Healthcare, 80*(2).

Hendricks, G., & Ludeman, K. (1997). *The corporate mystic: A guidebook for visionaries with their feet on the ground.* New York: Bantam.

Kouzes, J.M., & Posner, B.Z. (1995). *The leadership challenge: How to keep getting extraordinary things done in organizations (2nd ed.).* San Francisco: Jossey-Bass Press.

Kouzes, J.M., & Posner, B.Z. (1999). *Encouraging the heart: A leader's guide to rewarding and recognizing others.* San Francisco: Jossey-Bass Press.

Packer-Tursman, J. (1996). Reversing the revolving door syndrome. *Provider.*

Parsons, S., Parker, K.P., Ghose, R.P. (1998). Data strategies and benchmarks. *Journal of the Louisiana State Medical Society, 150,* 545–553.

Parsons, S.K, Simmons, W.P., Penn, K., & Furlough, M. (2003). Determinants of satisfaction and turnover among nursing assistants: The results of a statewide survey. *Journal of Gerontological Nursing.*

Schaefer, J.A., & Moos, R.H. (1996). Effects of work stressors and work climate on long-term-care staff's job morale and functioning. *Research in Nursing and Health, 19,* 63–73.

Whyte, D. (2002). *The heart aroused.* New York: Doubleday Press.

How Inspiration Affects Staff Members and Those for Whom They Care

"When you strengthen the life around you, perhaps you strengthen the life within you."
—Rachel Naomi Remen, from *My Grandfather's Blessings*

INTRODUCTION (15 minutes)

> **Tools Needed**
> - Flip chart
> - Markers

Have participants talk about a person that has inspired them the most in their lives.

Explain to participants what they should expect to learn from this module and list these expectations on the flip chart.
- Participants will have a better understanding of how inspiration can affect their lives.
- Participants will become more aware of not only who has inspired them the most but also why they were inspired.
- Participants will have an opportunity to share with each other how they have inspired those with whom they have worked.
- Participants will be able to recognize how inspiration can be a "mutual experience."

Ask participants if there are other expectations they would like to include, and write those on the flip chart.

WARM -UP EXERCISE (40 minutes)
Inspiration Matters

> **Tools Needed**
> - Flip chart
> - Markers
> - Poems, stories, or music that inspires the participants

Explain to participants that inspiration
- Can help them feel motivated, energized, hopeful, connected, and believed in
- Can be a way to help them connect to themselves and to one another
- Can make them more aware of how they touch others and how others can touch them
- Can help them feel good about themselves

Ask participants if they would like to add anything else.

Tell participants that the reason they were asked to bring in a poem, short story, or music was to be able to share with the group one way that they have been inspired.

Ask participants to listen carefully to each poem, quote, or story that is presented and think about the following:
- Did they find what was shared inspirational? Why or why not?
- What did they learn about the person sharing the piece?

Ask the person who is sharing the piece the following:
- Why did he or she share that particular piece?
- How does that piece inspire him or her?
- Could the person share the piece with the residents with whom he or she works?

CORE EXERCISE (30 minutes)
Inspiration Game

> **Tools Needed**
> - Posterboard with issues written on it
> - Masking tape
> - Markers, pens, and paper

Note: The trainer needs to have written one issue on each of the numbered poster boards, and then have them posted in each of the corners of the room. The issues that are to be written on the poster board are as follows:
- How can they inspire the elders with whom they work?
- How do the elders inspire them?
- When they are tired, stressed, and close to burnout, what or who might help the most to inspire them?

• How can inspiration help them with challenging residents?

Tell participants that they will be discussing one of four issues concerning inspiration. Separate participants into four groups, counting off by fours, and then have them go to the corner where that number is posted. For the next 10–15 minutes, they will discuss the issue associated with that number. One person from each group will need to record the group's key ideas to share with the larger group.

Walk around to each of the corners to make sure that the groups are able to come up with ideas. Give them about 10–15 minutes to process their ideas, and then bring them together to discuss their ideas with the larger group.

Ask each group to have one member state its question and report its ideas.

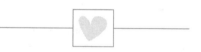

CLOSING (5 minutes)

Inquire if one of the participants would close the session with some inspirational words.

Ask participants to please fill out the evaluation form.

Evaluation Questions

1. Did you find this training helpful? (circle one)   Yes   No
    Please explain why or why not.

    _____

    _____

    _____

    _____

2. Will you be able to use the information you
    learned today at work? (circle one)   Yes   No

    _____

    _____

    _____

    _____

3. How can you feel more inspired in your work with the elders for whom you care?

    _____

    _____

    _____

    _____

4. Who inspires you the most at work? And why?

    _____

    _____

    _____

    _____

5. How did you feel after this workshop? (circle all that apply)

    good   encouraged   cared about
    sad   bored   listened to
    frustrated   informed   angry
    blessed   joyful   inspired
    motivated   good about myself

Spiritual Approaches to Caring for Elders

5

"If a man has two pennies, he should spend one
to buy a loaf of bread to sustain life and with the
other penny buy a flower to make a life worth living."
—A Chinese proverb

"Hope is the pillar of the world."
—Kanuri, from *A Tiny Treasury of African Proverbs*

OBJECTIVES

- To be able to define at least three reasons why a spiritual approach to care is important

- To become aware of how a spiritual approach to care affects the quality of caregiving

- To define the differences between a spiritual approach to care and a more traditional approach to care

ASSESSING THE SPIRITUAL NEEDS OF ELDERS

Caring for elders at the end of their lives can be both challenging and sacred. A spiritually-centered approach to care acknowledges that a person's spirit and soul are integral to the person. In addition, it offers elders hope at the end of life when they often feel hopeless. Cognitive and functional decline, along with dependency, can threaten the elder's sense of identity, connection to others, and meaning at the end of life. It can foster a loss of spirit. This is especially true and more prevalent among elders who live in nursing homes. Professionals working with elders in nursing homes struggle with how to preserve these individuals' well-being and spirit. Just providing for their physical needs denies them the opportunity to *finish well* and end their lives with meaning and dignity.

The research on how elders feel about their spirituality indicates that the older adult population is highly religious and spiritual. There is no evidence that the spirit succumbs to the aging process (Crowther, Parker, Achenbaum, Larimore, & Koenig, 2002; Isaia, Parker, & Murrow 1999; Kirkland & McIlveen 1998). Few articles discuss the importance of a spiritual approach to care, aside from making sure that residents have access to pastoral care and have the opportunity to participate in religious services. I believe teaching staff how to work with elders in a more spiritual way is extremely important.

In the past few years, there have been some encouraging studies regarding the importance of spirituality in maintaining quality of life. A number of articles have been published suggesting that professionals should begin to recognize the importance of evaluating the spiritual aspects of elders' lives. Although still considered new, this area is certainly gaining more attention (Koenig, 1999; Rowe & Kahn, 1997; Stuckey, 2001).

Much less research is available on spirituality in elders living in nursing homes or elders with dementia. There are some interesting reasons for this lack of attention to the spiritual assessment of elders in nursing homes.

1. Our culture has emphasized (until just recently) the medical model for caring for elders in nursing homes. This approach to care leaves little room for a spiritual focus of care. Our culture has painted a dim view of those elders who require nursing home care. They have supposedly come to the *end of the road*, with no hope. Those with dementia are considered by many to be *too far gone* to access the spiritual sides of themselves.

2. There has been concern among medical professionals about how to measure the effect of spirituality on elders who are frail. It can be difficult to evaluate this population, but several spirituality scales are currently being used to evaluate the higher-functioning population of elders:

    *   *The Spiritual Perspective Scale (SPS),* has been used by researchers in attempts to quantify spiritual viewpoints and activity of elders. This scale is based on a broad conceptualization of spirituality. Although it has been shown to be effective, there is some concern that this scale is not broad enough to capture spiritual perspectives that include all of the various philosophical and religious orientations (Touhy, 2001).

    *   *The Spirituality Index of Well-Being (SIWB)* has been found to be both reliable and valid in measuring subjective well-being in the elder population. Yet, there has not been much research on using this scale with nursing home residents (Daaleman, Frey, Wallace, & Studenski, 2002).

"In our daily lives, we must see that it is
not happiness that makes us grateful, but
gratefulness that makes us happy."
—Albert Clarke

THE EFFECT OF SPIRITUALITY ON SELF-ESTEEM

Because elders who lose their cognitive abilities often begin responding more
from their hearts, nursing home residents and elders with dementia are often
wonderful candidates for addressing issues of spirituality. In other words, the
things and people in their lives that have touched their heart continue to be
remembered and accessible. There are countless examples of elders who have vir-
tually no short-term and/or limited long-term memory but who can respond to
the religious sides of themselves. For example, many Christian elders can sing
every word of "Amazing Grace" or state the Lord's prayer without missing one
word; many Buddhist elders can remember meditations or chants, even when
they do not remember what they had for lunch just minutes after they have
eaten. Some elders continue to have a spiritual connection to nature, birds, butterflies, flowers, trees, and pets, and derive great comfort from these things—
comfort that is housed in the heart.

I will never forget the time I went to visit my mom at the nursing home in
which she was living and could not find her anywhere. When I asked where she
was, a staff member said, "I think she is in the chapel." I was surprised because
my mom was not religiously oriented, but, sure enough, when I went to the
chapel I found her sitting quietly. When I asked her why she was there, she said,
"I am praying to God to ask why I have Alzheimer's." I then asked my mom if she
would like to pray with me and she said, "Yes." The two of us sat together in the
synogogue and repeated the Shema, a sacred prayer, and asked God to help mom
feel safe and at peace. It was a moment I will always cherish. My experience with
my mother has reinforced my belief that a spiritual approach is highly effective
in working with nursing home elders and those with dementia.

The people, pets, meaningful life events, music, and foods that have fed my
mother's soul still live in her heart and are accessible to her. I am continually
touched by some of the comments she makes that clearly come from a spiritual
place inside her and by how much happiness the spiritual aspects of life bring to
her. An example that will always remain in my heart is my mother's strong connection to a music therapist, Tanya, who had worked with my mother when she
first entered the nursing home. Tanya was a special person in my mother's life.
Tanya and Mom had the strong connection of their love of music. My mother had
written songs for the piano, which she shared with Tanya when she was still able
to remember them and play them. Tanya and Mom would play together, Mom at
the piano and Tanya with the violin. They often performed for the residents and
staff at the nursing home. Their playing together filled my mother's soul and
moved her spirit. She was rarely depressed during the entire 3 years that Tanya
worked at the nursing home. Even after 9 years, whenever Tanya visited my

mother, her face just lit up and her spirit came alive! When Tanya no longer worked at the nursing home, Mom did not forget her! Although Mom's short- and long-term memory became quite impaired, and she had difficulty with completing sentences, when she saw Tanya, she clearly and with much emotion told her how much she loved her. I was not only touched by this relationship, but it reinforced for me the power of the memory of the heart and a person's spirit!

SPIRITUALITY AND SELF CARE

When elders lose their ability to manage their activities of daily living (the day-to-day things we all do to care for ourselves), they lose self-esteem and may even become resistant to accepting help. When they have dementia, they have the added challenge of not understanding why they need help.

A spiritual approach to activities of daily living care (ADLs) provides an important and meaningful way to support elders' sense of self-esteem. Furthermore, it is sometimes the only successful way to complete ADL care for that individual.

As a consultant, I often am asked by nursing homes directors to help with ADL challenges. I recall one situation in which a woman absolutely refused to take a bath. This behavior continued for weeks. The staff was frustrated, and her family was becoming upset with the staff. I was consulted to provide some suggestions. After spending some time with her and reading her social history, I found out that she loved to dance and sing. She even had specific songs that she enjoyed singing over and over again. I suggested to the caregivers that they learn those songs and then "dance and sing her" to the bathroom and through the entire bath. This approach was successful, not only because the woman was able to successfully complete taking a bath but also because both the caregiver and resident enjoyed the experience of singing and dancing together.

Another situation involved a gentleman who had dementia and consistently refused to let the staff help him to dress. He wanted to stay in his robe and pajamas all day. Again, I was consulted to provide some suggestions. After spending time with him and reading his social history, I found out that he was a very religious man. He was an elder in his church and taught a bible class for years. I suggested to the caregivers that when they were ready to help dress him that they tell him that he needed to get dressed for church and engage him in a discussion of what it was like being an elder and teaching bible class. It worked almost every time. Sometimes they would sing hymns together while dressing him. The experience proved to be meaningful for him and the caregivers.

IMPORTANCE OF SPIRITUALITY GROUPS

In addition to the powerful ways that one-to-one spiritual approaches to care can provide for staff and elders, a group approach could be another way to encourage a meaningful experience and to help elders feel good about themselves. I smile when I remember a spirituality group I was conducting with a group of elders who had dementia. We were sitting in a circle sharing our feelings about what we were grateful for. One 83-year-old woman responded by saying she was grateful for her mama and daddy, whom she loved and who still cared about her. Her parents had been deceased for more than 25 years. Yet, it was clear by the look on her face and her tone of voice that she believed they were still alive. The lady sitting next to her in the circle responded to her by saying with a tone of amazement, "Are they still living?" "Yes," she retorted rather emphatically. "Oh, how wonderful," said the lady next to her. I thought this was a great exchange of spiritual energy and feelings!

I will never forget the look on an elder woman's face during another one of my spirituality groups sessions. This resident was not able to speak English anymore. She had reverted to her childhood language of Russian. She also carried a teddy bear that she clearly thought was her baby. She had a tendency to pace and would walk up and down the hallways holding her "baby." While gathering the elders for the group, I asked her to join in. Staff warned me that she would only stay for a minute and then wander off. Once everyone had been seated, I asked the group members what they felt blessed about. I turned to her first and said, "I bet you feel blessed to have your baby?" She looked at me with a big smile on her face and shook her head "yes." She stayed with me throughout the entire group, smiling down at her baby, and gracing us with her gentle spirit.

There is no doubt that spirituality groups are a wonderful way to access the spirit and reinforce meaning for elders, no matter how impaired people are. Every activity program for elders should offer a wide range of spiritual activities and groups, not just religious services. And for those with dementia, accessing the spiritual sides of these elders can provide peace and comfort.

ENCOURAGING THE SPIRIT OF THE STAFF

In addition to nurturing the spirit of the elder, encouraging the spirit of staff members who care for elders is equally important. In *The Caring Spirit* workshops, I often ask staff, "Have you brought your spirits to work? Are you caring for elders from that spiritual and heartfelt place?" When staff members care for elders in a spiritual way, they think about taking care of the elders' spirits and souls, not just their disabilities or diseases. It is important to consider the whole person, not just the tasks that need to be completed. Approaching care in a spiritual way allows opportunities to engage with elders in a deeper and more satisfying way. It fosters a *mutual* caring as the hearts of both the elder and the staff member are interconnected. Staff members who provide care in a spiritual way foster kindness, compassion, gratitude, and integrity.

Most staff working in long-term care are very open to a spiritual approach to care. When asked how they cope with some of the challenges of their work, staff members often share that they pray before they go to work or ask a higher power for patience, courage, and strength to support them through their day. They mention singing hymns, saying prayers, or meditating with many of the elders with whom they care. In thinking about their responses and observing the relationships they have with elders, it is important to help staff members recognize this work as *sacred*. When caring comes from a sacred place, loving kindness and compassion flow easily.

The focus of Training Module 5 is to help participants become more aware of the differences between a spiritual approach to care and a more traditional approach to care, and how a more spiritual approach can affect care.

REFERENCES

Crowther, M.R., Parker, M.W., Achenbaum, W.W., Larimore, W.L., & Koenig, H.G. (2002). Rowe and Kahn's model of successful aging revisted: Positive spirituality—The forgotten factor. *The Gerontologist, 42*(5).

Daaleman, T.P., Frey, B.B., Wallace, D., & Studenski, S.A. (2002). Spirituality index of well-being scale: Development and testing of a new measure. *The Journal of Family Practice, 51*(11).

Isaia, D., Parker, V., & Murrow, E. (1999). Spiritual well-being among older adults. *Journal of Gerontological Nursing, 25*(8), 15–21.

Kirkland, K.H., & McIlveen, H. (1998). *Full circle: Spiritual therapy for the elderly.* New York: Hayworth Press.

Koenig, H.G. (1999). *The healing power of faith.* New York: Simon & Schuster Press.

Rowe, J.W., & Kahn, R.L. (1997). Successful aging. *The Gerontologist, 37,* 433–440.

Stuckey, J.C. (2001). Blessed assurance: The role of religion and spirituality in Alzheimer's disease caregivers and other significant life events. *Journal of Aging Studies, 15,* 69–84.

Touhy, T.A. (2001). Nurturing hope and spirituality in the nursing home. *Holistic Nursing Practice, 15*(4), 45–46.

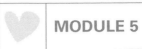 **MODULE 5**

Spiritual Approaches to Caring for Elders

"It is better to be loved than feared."
—Senegal, from *A Tiny Treasury of African Proverbs*

INTRODUCTION (15 minutes)

> **Tools Needed**
> • Flip chart
> • Markers

 Have participants introduce themselves. Read the quote from the beginning of this module to participants. Ask them what they think it means in the context of providing a spiritual approach to care.

 Explain to participants what objectives they should expect to learn from this module and list these on the flip chart.
- Participants will learn to be more spiritual in their approach to care.
- Participants will learn how a spiritual approach differs from a more traditional approach to care.
- Participants will learn how a spiritual approach to caring affects how they feel about themselves and the elders for whom they care.

 Ask participants if there are other expectations they would like to include, and write those on the flip chart.

WARM-UP EXERCISE (30 minutes)
Catching the Heart and Spirit of Caring

> **Tools Needed**
> • Hershey kisses

 Explain to participants that they will engage in a simple game. The game reinforces a spiritual way of caring. They will have an opportunity to share an example of how they spiritually work with elders. Each participant will have the opportunity to *catch a kiss* that is thrown to him or her. Once a person catches a Hershey kiss and shares an example, he or she will throw a Hershey kiss to another participant, until everyone has had a chance to share. Before starting the game, share with participants some ways they might have cared for elders using a spiritual approach. Some examples include

- Shared humor and laughs
- Provided hugs and touch
- Brought in stuffed animals for elders to hold and hug
- Sang songs with elders
- Danced with elders
- Prayed with elders
- Recited bible passages
- Used a gentle and/or calm approach
- Shared a compassionate exchange

 Ask participants what they learned about their approach to caring. Did this exercise help them to think about some different ways of caring?

CORE EXERCISE (40 minutes)
The Prescription Bottle

Tools Needed
- Handouts 5.1 and 5.2
- Pens

 Explain to the participants that this exercise will help them to understand the difference between a spiritual approach and a traditional approach to caring. They will learn how their approach directly affects the caregiving experience.

 Inform the participants that they will work with two *prescription bottles*. One bottle is filled with pills, which, when taken by the elder, cause him or her to experience care in a spiritual way. The other bottle is filled with pills, which, when taken by the elder, cause the elder to experience care in a traditional way. Participants are to write down the *side effects* of the pills from each bottle, good or bad.

 Have participants divide into small groups. One person from each group should serve as the recorder. The group members will decide together what side effects would result from each bottle of pills. After they have listed all of the side effects, they will read them to the entire group.

Note: Handout 5.1 lists the contents of each pill bottle. The participants will also have Handout 5.2 on which they will write out the spiritual and traditional side effects.

 Ask participants to share one new *side effect* or difference that they learned when comparing a spiritual approach to care versus a traditional approach to care.

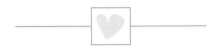

CLOSING (5 minutes)

 Thank participants for being willing to participate in the training and ask them to complete the evaluation form.

Evaluation Questions

1. Did you find this training helpful? (circle one)   Yes   No
   Please explain why or why not.

   _____

   _____

   _____

   _____

2. Will you be able to use the information
   you learned today at work? (circle one)   Yes   No
   If yes, give at least two examples.

   _____

   _____

   _____

   _____

3. What is the difference between a spiritual approach versus
   a traditional approach to caring? Give at least three examples.

   _____

   _____

   _____

   _____

4. Why might a spiritual approach to care help you enjoy your work more?

   _____

   _____

   _____

   _____

5. How did you feel after this workshop? (circle all that apply)

good	encouraged	cared about
sad	bored	listened to
frustrated	informed	angry
blessed	joyful	inspired
motivated	good about myself	

Prescription Bottle Ingredients

What's in the Spiritual prescription bottle

- Approaching the elder slowly
- Showing respect by not talking *over* the person
- Thinking about the person as a *soul*
- Showing patience and understanding
- Taking time when giving care
- Feeling compassion for the person
- Listening
- Encouraging independence
- Showing your spiritual side to the elder
- Distracting by singing, praying, and dancing

What's in the Traditional prescription bottle

- Getting the task done
- Hurrying the person along, as you have others to care for
- Not being too concerned about how the elder feels
- Not listening because you don't have the time
- Talking about residents because they can't hear or they won't understand
- Discouraging independence, as it is too much of a bother
- Caring for the person's disease or handicap rather than caring about the person
- Trying not to feel, just doing the job
- Not showing your spiritual side because it won't matter or there isn't time

Prescription Bottle Side Effects

Write down each *side effect* from the spiritual and traditional pill bottles. Look at the list of ingredients in the spiritual and traditional prescription bottles (Handout 5.1) and try to write a side effect that corresponds to each item.

Spiritual Side Effects	Traditional Side Effects

How Staff Members Can Find Support within the Work They Do

"...each of us may have left far more
behind us than we may ever know."
—Rachel Naomi Remen, from *My Grandfather's Blessings*

OBJECTIVES

- To increase awareness among leadership of the importance of changing the culture of caring in the work environment

- To show the value of helping staff members understand and recognize the many ways to find strength in the work they do

- To help leadership teach staff how to ask for help and support

HOW LONG-TERM CARE STAFF IS VALUED

Staff workers in long-term care have long been exploited, criticized, de-valued, and not recognized for the hard work they perform. The media has been quick to focus on the worst-case examples and has found information that supports those cases. An *us against them* attitude toward long-term care staff is pervasive. Although a small percentage of staff members are not providing high-quality care, the majority of caregivers and other nursing staff are, and they have entered the field because they view this work as *a calling*.

Researchers Wrzesniewski, et. al. (1997), in a study about how workers view their jobs, identified three distinct categories. In the first category, the worker views his or her job as simply a job. The focus is on the financial rewards that the job brings. The nature of the work may hold little interest, pleasure, or fulfillment. In the second category, workers view their jobs as a career. The primary focus is on advancement. They chose their jobs because prestige, social status, and power motivate them. There may be more personal investment, but only if the promotions continue. In the third category, workers see their jobs as a way to contribute to society. They tend to love what they do and are less motivated by money than by satisfaction in helping others.

This research is particularly interesting because it suggests the importance of learning about why people choose the type of work they do. I have always believed that most caregivers in long-term care select this work out of a passion for it, not because they desire prestige, power, or money. It has been my experience that most caregivers who work in long-term care accept these jobs with positive intentions. Unfortunately, I also believe that the system or the hardships that accompany these jobs encourage staff to lose spirit because:

- The physical environments in which they work are depressing

- Training and consistent supervision are lacking

- Understaffing makes staff caseloads extremely difficult to manage and still provide quality care

- Resources are inadequate

- Wages are low and caregivers often have to work second jobs

- The incidence of staff injuries is high

- Management and society in general do not value this work

- Staff members are not encouraged to take care of themselves

These are just a sample of reasons why staff are not performing at their optimal capacity. I have traveled the country, providing supervision, consultation, and training to staff in long-term care. I hear the same concerns from staff everywhere I go, and the research around staffing concerns echoes their responses. Staff members feel underpaid, undervalued, and neglected (Packer-Tursman, 1996; Schaefer & Moos, 1996; Lin, Yin, & Li, 2002). In order to create a culture that cares, we must value these workers and help them to find continued strength for the work they do.

Multitudes of caregivers manifest love, compassion, and genuine caring toward elders. Many caregivers continue to work in awful work situations and place their health on the line simply because they care about the elders for whom they are responsible.

VIEWING LONG-TERM CARE THROUGH A DIFFERENT LENS

In the next 20 years, with the onslaught of baby boomers entering their elder years, there will be a great need to provide resources and support for this age cohort. We need to be proactive about how we are going to provide services to this large group of elders.

As a baby boomer myself, I am very concerned about what my future elder years will look like. I know I want to live in a culture that cares. I also know I do not want to live out my later years in the type of long-term care environments we currently have available. As Dr. Bill Thomas, creator of The Eden Alternative, so bluntly states, "There are only two populations we institutionalize, elders and prisoners."

Long-term care leaders must brainstorm, think outside of the box, and be willing to stop perpetuating the current conditions in long-term care. The following are some suggestions for leadership to think about:

1. **Leadership must change the way people think about growing old and what it means to be an elder in our country.**

   - An inspirational program has been developed called Aging to Saging based on the work of Zalman Schachter-Shalomi and Ronald Miller. They contend that leadership needs to create a meaningful role and place in our society for our elders. They believe that role is one of *sage*. Many institutions and organizations have embraced this philosophy, yet it is still very much in its infancy. Along with creating a meaningful role and title for elders, we need to stop thinking of them as *burdens* to our society. As long as we continue to view them in this negative way, we will continue to perpetuate negative stereotypes that de-value elders in our society.

2. **Leadership needs to think about the later stage of life as a sacred stage of life.**

   - Defining this stage as sacred offers a different perspective on thinking about those who work with elders. We can see the jobs that care staff perform along with other professionals in long-term care as sacred work.

   - Thinking about the later stage of life as sacred leads to thinking outside of the box. It causes leadership to ask the question, "What might be a way to frame the role of caregiver and create deeper meaning and connection for the person in that role?" One way to do this is to compare caregivers to angels. It is important to point out how *angelic* traits provide ways to help workers cope with the many challenges of their work through strength, hope, courage, and inspiration.

3. **Leadership must follow the example of the Pioneer Network (PN),** a national organization that is attempting to bring attention to this area and to create positive change in the long-term care industry. The PN recognizes the importance of changing the culture in long-term care toward a more positive culture for elders and those who work in it. It has been seeking out professionals and organizations that are committed to positive change with a strong emphasis toward valuing the later stage of life. Since the PN has been in existence, it has grown and sparked some attention. However, there is much left to be done.

A UNIQUE PERSPECTIVE ON ANGELS

Historically, angels have always existed. In examining recorded history, images of angels have appeared throughout Western culture and cultures around the world. In *The Everything Angels Book,* author M.J. Abadie examined the research written about angels and their origins. As she examined ancient history, she found that many cultures, including the Egyptians, Greeks, Persians, Assyrians, and Mesopotamians, acknowledged winged beings.

The term *angel* was not officially used until the formation of the Christian and Jewish religions. Frequent references to angels exist in the Bible, both from the Old and New Testaments. The Bible translates the word *angel* as "messenger of God." The New Testament offers images of angels that are more personalized, as friends to human beings. In this context, angels are seen as powerful spirits that can be called on to help humans through difficult times.

The Koran also contains images and stories about angels, while the Hindu religion has a version of angels called *Feresh'ta,* which are winged spiritual counselors. A similar image is seen in the Native American culture in the Black Elk, viewed as a mysterious healer.

Roots for the word angel—in Latin, Greek, and Sanskrit—translate similarly as either "divine spirit," "courier," or "messenger" (Abadie, 2000). Two of the most common ways angels were physically described in her research were

- A form through which a specific essence or energy force can be transmitted for a specific purpose

- Celestial beings of pure light that vibrate at very high rates which often make them invisible to the eye

Abadie noted that physical descriptions of angels seemed fairly similar and that all angels seemed to have wings. It seems that the wings of angels communicate power, grace, and an alert readiness to move at God's injunction. Furthermore, she found that angels came in many forms and that how people perceived them depended on their own personal belief systems and what images they received as children.

In our society, many people believe only in things they can see and touch. Thus, they exercise much caution around the topic of angels. Others have embraced the concept of *angel* because it is a part of their religious beliefs. It seems most people believe at least in the emotional definition of angels. There are many positive references to angels in our language:

"That child is a little angel."

"You are such an angel for doing that."

"Only an angel could have been behind this."

"What a precious angel you are to me."

In addition, references to angels abound in movies, on television, and in books.

In today's society, angels are looked on as sources of strength and courage, providers of support, and messengers of hope. They impart special graces such as beauty, love, kindness, and comfort. They brighten the world and spread joy. Whether one truly believes in angels as spirits or beings does not really matter. What is important is that in today's society angels are cherished and the concept of *angel* is given great meaning.

Often, the word angel is reserved for the special things people do for one another or for how one feels about a special person. Many people have a *guardian angel,* someone special who has inspired them, unconditionally loved them, comforted them, nurtured and supported them, and guided them through the journeys of their lives.

Most people have experienced an *angelic moment,* when they have witnessed the birth of a child, a shooting star, a beautiful rainbow, a person's last breath, or a close call with death. These experiences help many of us to truly believe we were "touched by an angel."

Training Module 6 was created to recognize the tremendous work done by people who care for and about elders in their day-to-day lives, and to help caregivers realize and appreciate what they do as "angel like." In this module, participants will learn and understand

- How the work they do is "angel like"

- How they can find the strength within themselves to do this special kind of work

- How to find strength externally, from each other, and from other sources

REFERENCES

Abadie, M.J. (2000). *The everything angels book: Discover the guardians, messengers, and heavenly companions in your life.* Holbrook, MA: Adams Media Corp.

Lama, D., & Cutler, H.C. *The art of happiness at work.* New York: Riverhead Books.

Lin, S., Yin, T.J.C., Li, I. (2002) An exploration of work stressors and correlators for nurse's aides in long-term-care facilities. *Journal of Nursing Research,10*(3).

Packer-Tursman, J. (February, 1996). Reversing the revolving door syndrome. *Provider.*

Schachter-Shalomi, Z., & Miller, R.S. (1995). *From aging to saging: A profound new vision of growing older.* New York: Warner Books.

Schaefer, J.A., & Moos, R.H. (1996). Effects of work stressors and work climate on long-term care staff's job morale and functioning. *Research in Nursing and Health, 19,* 63-73.

Wrzesniewski, A., McCauley, C.R., Rozin, P., & Schwartz, B. (1997). Jobs, careers, and callings: People's relations to their work. *Journal of Research in Personality, 31,* 21-33.

| MODULE 6 |

How Staff Members Can Find Support within the Work They Do

"Service is always a work of the heart."
—Rachel Naomi Remen, from *My Grandfather's Blessings*

Introduction (10 minutes)

> **Tools Needed**
> • Flip chart
> • Markers

ask

Have participants introduce themselves and then ask them the following question: "Who or what in their lives has provided them with the most strength?"

explain

Explain to participants what they should expect to learn from this module and list these expectations on the flip chart.
- Participants will be able to identify some of the ways they are like angels.
- Participants will learn different ways to draw strength from each other and from outside sources.
- Participants will experience how to tap into the multiple sources of strength they have within themselves.

ask

Ask participants if there are other expectations they would like to include, and write those on the flip chart.

WARM- UP EXERCISE (25 minutes)

> **Tools Needed**
> • Flip chart
> • Markers
> • Handout 6.1

Note: Share some of the information from the beginning of the chapter about angels before asking participants to complete Handout 6.1.

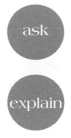

Have participants separate into groups of two or three. Give the participants the handout with questions they are to ask one another.

Explain to the participants that you will first read the questions to them and provide examples to help them get started. The questions from the handout and some suggested answers follow:

1. What are some of the traits that angels possess?

    Suggestions might include
    - Integrity
    - Support
    - Love
    - Caring
    - Kindness
    - Strength
    - Nurturing
    - Courage
    - Understanding
    - Hope
    - Guardian
    - Inspiration

2. What "angel like" traits do you see in yourselves?

    Prompts include
    - Are some of the above words ways they might define themselves as "angel like"?
    - Are there traits they learned from their parents/grandparents, aunts/uncles, and so forth?

3. How might you be more "angel like" as care providers to elders?

    - Explore possible barriers to being more "angel like" in their work.
    - Suggest finding ways to be less hurried, more patient; to spend time listening to and getting to know the elders; and to share more of themselves and their spiritual sides.

In their small groups, ask participants to take 10 minutes to share their comments with each other. Explain to them that after they share with each other in their small groups, they will come together as one group and share some of their comments.

Note: During these 10 minutes, walk around and assist any participants who need it. Let the group know when their 10 minutes are up.

Have participants share comments from one of the three questions. Write the answers on the flip chart so the group can see them.

"Unless someone like you cares a whole awful lot,
Nothing is going to get better, it's not."
—Dr. Seuss, from *The Lorax*

CORE EXERCISE (35 minutes)
Ask the Angels

> **Tools Needed**
> - Flip chart
> - Markers
> - Handout 6.2 (copy and cut out the set of Angel Cards in this handout)
> - A box for the Angel Cards

Explain to participants that this exercise will help them explore some of their own strengths, talents, and inner resources.

Ask participants to think about the following suggestions to help them recognize their strengths, talents, and inner resources:

1. Think about situations in which they had to be strong in their work or personal lives. Examples might include

   - When they lost a parent at a young age and had to help raise their siblings
   - When they went through a difficult divorce
   - When they lost a job
   - When they had to care for an ailing parent or grandparent
   - When they had to care for an elder who was very agitated and lashed out
   - When they lost a child

2. Have them ask close friends, co-workers, or supervisors what their strengths are and what they think their talents might be. Asking for feedback can provide another way of seeing themselves.

3. Participants can pay attention to what gives them joy, satisfaction, and love in their lives. They can also pay attention to how people seem to respond to them. Do people appear to enjoy their company, smile when they see them, joke with them, want to hug them, tell them they love and appreciate them?

Ask participants how often they feel exhausted or worn out?
- Do they feel like they give more than they receive?
- Do they feel their work situations or life situations make it hard for them to tap into their strengths, inner resources, or talents?
- Do they feel burned out?

Explain to participants that providing care to elders can be draining. Bringing spirituality into their lives could be one important way to replenish themselves. Also explain to the participants that this exercise can provide alternative ways to gather courage and hope. It will help them understand their own strengths, talents, and inner resources. However, remind them that they do not have to participate in this exercise if they choose not to do so.

Once you have gone over the above questions, give each participant a chance to pick one card out of the Angel Card box. Before the participants pick a card, they are to silently ask the angels what they might need to help them care better for themselves or for the elders they work with. They can decide what question they want to ask the angels. After they pick a card, they can choose to share the card they picked with the group and think about why they received that particular card; they can also just keep their thoughts to themselves.

Explain to participants that you will be asking them how the card they picked might apply to their lives.

For example, if they picked the card *understanding,* the trainer might ask them why they received that card now? Ask them to explore some reasons, such as:

- Do they need to be more understanding in their lives with their spouses, children, elders, or themselves?
- Are the angels encouraging them to continue being understanding in their lives, as it helps them cope with some of the challenges they face?

If they picked the card *honesty,* why might they have needed that card now? Ask them to explore some reasons, such as:

- Do they need to be more honest with themselves, their co-workers, or boss?
- Are the angels encouraging them to continue to be honest in their lives, as it serves them best?

Note: This exercise can elicit a variety of emotions and feelings for the participants. It is important to allow the participants time to experience their emotions.

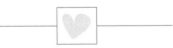

Closing (5 minutes)

Thank the participants for being willing to participate in the training and ask them to fill out the evaluation form.

Evaluation Questions

1. Did you find this training helpful? (circle one)   Yes   No
   Please explain why or why not.

   _____
   _____
   _____
   _____

2. What angelic traits do you think you have after participating in this workshop?
   List at least three.

   _____
   _____
   _____
   _____

3. How do you think you have been like an angel to the elders for whom you care?

   _____
   _____
   _____
   _____

4. How did you feel after this workshop? (circle all that apply)

good	encouraged	cared about
sad	bored	listened to
frustrated	informed	angry
blessed	joyful	inspired
motivated	good about myself	

Questions to Ponder:
Being Angel-like

1. What "angel like" traits do you see in yourselves?

    _____
    _____
    _____
    _____
    _____
    _____
    _____
    _____

2. How might you be more "angel like" as care providers to elders?

    _____
    _____
    _____
    _____
    _____
    _____
    _____

3. What angel traits do you use when providing care to elders?

    _____
    _____
    _____
    _____
    _____
    _____
    _____

Angel Cards
(Copy and cut apart)

forgiveness	obedience	purification	light
education	love	freedom	simplicity
faith	joy	expectancy	inspiration
delight	responsibility	creativity	openness
surrender	release	beauty	truth
healing	clarity	honesty	sisterhood/ brotherhood
courage	gratitude	enthusiasm	transformation
trust	purpose	responsibility	play
flexibility	willingness	understanding	grace
patience	power	synthesis	integrity
strength	humor	efficiency	communication
birth	compassion	abundance	harmony
balance	adventure	peace	spontaneity
			tenderness

Spiritual Ways to Cope with Stress

> "Only by connecting with the nature of the spirit can we realize that all problems and negativity in the world are just situations in which we decide what we want to make of them."
> —John Morton, from *The Blessings Already Are*

OBJECTIVES

- To highlight the importance of recognizing the way stress affects long-term care staff interpersonally

- To demonstrate the opportunities available to staff members when they use their spiritual sides to cope with the stress of their jobs

- To teach spiritual coping tools to leadership

UNDERSTANDING STRESS AND CAREGIVING

Researchers have provided strong evidence implicating stress as an important factor in high turnover, low morale, and poor job satisfaction among long-term care workers. Complicating matters, there is great concern about whether there will be enough staff to care for the 20% increase in the population of elders projected by 2020. It is projected that there will be a critical shortage in the next decade (Fitzpatrick, 2002). The lack of available staff adds another layer of stress to the current struggle with high turnover and with finding and retaining staff. In the majority of nursing homes, the turnover rate of direct care staff ranges from 50% to 100% (Parsons, Simmons, Penn, & Furlough, 2003). In addition, The U.S. Department of Labor indicates that long-term care facilities are among the fastest-growing industries in the nation (Bureau of Labor Statistics, 1997–1998).

The following are some key issues mentioned in the research on caregiver stress and its effect on long-term care (Remsburg, Armacost, & Bennett, 1999; Schaefer & Moos, 1996; Will, 1997):

- Stress is greater in settings that require intense physical and cognitive care of the elders.

- Stress is greater when the staff workload is too high.

- Stress is greater in environments in which supervisors provide little support and supervision of staff.

- Stress is greater in caregivers who feel their work is not valued and appreciated by management or by the elders' families.

- Stress is greater in staff who feel they are not respected for their skills and are not involved in the decision-making process.

- Stress is greater in staff who feel they cannot spend enough time with the elders for whom they care.

These key issues will not surprise most long-term care professionals, particularly those who are direct care workers. Yet it seems that we, as leaders, are still "missing the boat" in helping staff cope most effectively with their stress.

A DIFFERENT PERSPECTIVE ON STRESS AND CAREGIVING

Despite all my professional knowledge and experience, my strong friend and family support network, and the influence of a caring nursing home, I still felt a great deal of stress and sadness in my role as caregiver with my mother. I searched for the "missing link" to caregiving by observing staff and searching in my own heart for ways to cope with the stress of being my mother's caregiver. Then, I attended a powerful workshop on "Spirituality and Aging" and had a profound experience with the keynote speaker, Ram Dass. He spoke from his heart about his spiritual journey toward finding ways to cope with the stress of living through a serious stroke. I was so inspired by his presentation that I read his book, *Still Here,* and watched his documentary entitled *Fierce Grace.* Those two sources helped me realize I had not explored all of the spiritual options available to me that might offer some different perspectives and new ways of coping.

In 2001, my spiritual journey began. Since then, I have opened myself to the myriad ways I can experience my spirituality at its fullest. I have noticed that I not only experience less stress and sadness, but also believe I am coping much more effectively with my mother's disease. For example, I have exposed myself to as many teachings of different spiritual faiths as possible, keeping a willingness to stay open and nonjudgmental. I have found a great deal of comfort in each of them, deriving the most comfort in Eastern teachings and Native American Indian beliefs and teachings. I also have explored how nature can help me to find peace and comfort with my life challenges. I have chosen to work in macro photography (i.e., close-up photography). When I feel stressed, I spend time connecting to and photographing flowers and other creations of nature. This therapeutic hobby helps me to slow down, be more observant, and find ways to connect. I have been enjoying gardening and how my connection with the earth refreshes and replenishes my spirit. I make sure I allow myself time to *just be,* whether it is relaxing to music, taking a walk in the park, or soaking in a warm, bubbly bath when I feel stressed. These activities quickly calm me and slow down my breathing so I can relax.

I began to share stories of how I was expanding my relationship to spirituality both personally and professionally. In doing so, I started asking staff members to comment on my stories and then to share their own stories. Contrary to what one might think since spirituality is very personal, I found most staff felt quite comfortable in sharing their spiritual sides and stories. Many even acknowledged how helpful it was for them to do so. I will never forget one story that a staff member shared. She mentioned that she had worked with elders who have dementia for more than 20 years. She shared how she was able to care for a resident who became very agitated when staff tried to put her to bed at night. She said that no one could get this resident to sleep, thus the resident would walk the halls at night, crying, and sometimes screaming. Eventually the resident would be given medication. When this staff member was assigned to that resident and was getting ready to put the resident to sleep, the staff member sat on the bed with her, put her arms around her, and rocked and sang to her. She sang old hymns and spiritual songs that she knew the resident was familiar with. She remarked that she never had trouble getting her to sleep. As I listened to her story and envisioned her singing and rocking this dear elder to sleep, I had tears in my eyes. I looked around at all the staff members and they, too, were profoundly touched. What struck me was how effective this simple act of spiritual kindness was. The resident was less agitated and able to go to bed calmly and peacefully, and the staff member was able to prevent a very stressful experience for herself. In utilizing spiritual coping tools, she created a spiritual experience that was soothing to both of them! This story paved the way for many discussions around helping the staff utilize spiritual coping tools when working in stressful conditions.

Training Module 7 was created to help participants identify some of the opportunities they have to nourish their souls and spirits at work and find healthier ways to cope with job stress.

REFERENCES

Dass, R. (2000). *Still here: Embracing aging, changing and dying.* New York: Riverhead Press.

Fitzpatrick, P.G. (2002). Turnover of certified nursing assistants: A major problem for long-term care facilities. *Hospital Topics. 80*(2).

Kornfield, J. (1993). *A path with heart: A guide through the perils and promises of spiritual life.* New York: Bantam.

Parsons, S.K., Simmons, W.P., Penn, K., & Furlough, M. (2003). Determinants of satisfaction and turnover among nursing assistants: The results of a statewide survey. *Journal of Gerontological Nursing.*

Remsburg, R.E., Armacost, K.A., & Bennett, R.G. (1999). Improving nursing assistant turnover and stability rates in a long-term-care facility. *Geriatric Nurse Management, 20*(4).

Schaefer, J.A., & Moos, R.H. (1996). Effects of work stressor and work climate on long-term care staff's job morale and functioning. *Research in Nursing and Health 19,* 63–73.

Will, K.E. (December, 1999). Tactics for reducing certified nursing assistant turnover. *Provider.*

| **MODULE 7** | # Spiritual Ways to Cope with Stress

"A sense of humor can help you overlook the unattractive, tolerate the unpleasant, cope with the unexpected, and smile through the un-bearable."
—Moshe Waldoks

INTRODUCTION (15 minutes)

Tools Needed
- Flip chart
- Markers
- Index cards
- Pens

ask

Have participants introduce themselves. Give participants an index card and ask them write down one work situation they find stressful. Let them know that those situations will be used later in a training exercise. Pick up the index cards to use later in the training.

explain

Share with participants what they should expect to learn from this module and list these objectives on the flip chart.
- Participants will be able to identify what opportunities they have to *nourish their souls.*
- Participants will learn how to *nourish their souls.*
- Participants will understand how a spiritual approach to stress can be helpful in coping.
- Participants will learn some spiritual tools to help them cope with stress at work.

ask

Ask participants if there are other expectations they would like to include, and write those on the flip chart.

WARM-UP EXERCISE (45 minutes)
Spirituality and Stress—Why Not?

> **Tools Needed**
> - Flip chart
> - Markers
> - Index cards that participants filled out
> - Basket to hold index cards
> - Handout 7.1

ask

Ask participants how they define stress. Write their comments on the flip chart. You might want to add some additional ways to define stress such as:
- Stress creates situations when we feel emotionally, physically, or spiritually out of sync.
- We often will have symptoms that are upsetting or uncomfortable. We might become agitated, sad, easily frustrated, depressed, anxious, angry, and overwhelmed. We might also exhibit discomfort in different parts of our bodies. We could develop headaches, stomach distress, backaches, skin rashes, twitches in our eyes, and so forth.
- Stress can prevent us from conducting ourselves in healthy ways. At work, we might call out sick, come in late, not complete our work, take out our anger on a resident or other staff member, and lose spirit and passion for our work.
- Stress can cause us to unintentionally harm the elders we are caring for, or other staff members, or ourselves. We may neglect or abuse a resident, we may become verbally abusive to a staff member, or we may take our stress out on ourselves by overeating, drinking alcohol, taking drugs, and so forth.
- Recognizing stress as a warning sign can actually help us take better care of ourselves—if we listen to the warning signs before they get out of control!

explain

Explain to participants that they will learn some spiritual approaches to stress that they can apply at work. Following are some thoughts to ponder about spiritual aspects of coping with stress:
- Be aware of how stress might be getting in the way of connecting to your heart. If you let your *head* take over, you tend to react. This can result in being more explosive, angry, and even abusive. If you can stay in your *heart*, you are better able to find ways of coping that involve compassion, patience, and understanding toward yourself and others.
- Be aware of how stress can block you from understanding how the other person may be feeling. It is not unusual for us to feel disconnected from how another person is feeling when we are consumed with our own distress. When we are feeling "stressed out" it is even more impor-

tant to take a step back and consider whether our stress is preventing us from connecting to others or allowing others to help us.

- Be able to place yourself in another person's shoes. It is important to recognize how stress affects others as well. Remember that when people feel stressed out, it is not unusual for them to take out their feelings on you. Try not to take what they are saying or how they are behaving toward you personally. When you are in a spiritual place, you are able to be compassionate, and can place yourself in their shoes. You listen from your heart and acknowledge that you are hearing how stressed out or upset they are! This practice certainly takes time to master and is not always easy to do, especially if the person is attacking you or if the situation stirs up your emotions too. When you are able to stay spiritually connected, however, it becomes easier to let go and be less reactive.

- Learn not to make assumptions and be willing to open yourself up to new ways of thinking. Stressful situations can cause you to be reactive, which tends to place you in a judgmental position. When you make assumptions, you shut down possibilities. When you cope with stress in a more spiritual way, you put aside your judgments and, instead of reacting, you stay open and willing to hear another person's side of the situation. You see *the opportunities* in the situation.

explain Explain to participants that they will now have the opportunity to practice seeing stressful situations from a different perspective.

ask Ask participants to listen to the following example and try to think about what it might feel like to be in either *co-worker A's* or *co-worker B's* shoes.

explain Explain to participants that they will have a chance to discuss this activity together after you share the scenario. Give them Handout 7.1 so they can read along with the trainer if they like.

Scenario

Co-worker A has not been feeling well. She has been very tired because her baby daughter has been cutting new teeth and has been keeping her from getting enough sleep for several days. She finds herself less patient and more easily angered than usual. She knows that she is taking her frustration out on *co-worker B,* but has not been able to do anything about it because she feels so stressed out. In the meantime, *co-worker B* has been very frustrated to the point of being angry with *co-worker A,* as she has not been pulling her load. *Co-worker A* also tends to make excuses and never apologizes for not doing her job. *Co-worker B* has had it; she feels stressed out and angry and finally yells at *co-worker A.* The two co-workers end up having a loud verbal argument in front of several residents.

Have participants think first about *co-worker A's* situation. Tell them to place themselves in *co-worker A's* shoes. How could both workers connect to their hearts and souls so they could handle this situation in a spiritual rather than a stressful way? Ask participants to answer the following questions:

1. How could you identify with *co-worker A's* situation more from the heart?
2. What questions would you ask *co-worker A* so you might understand her situation better?
3. What characteristics would you need if you were to approach her in a more spiritual way? Examples might include the following:
    *   Understanding
    *   Patience
    *   Compassion
    *   Gentleness
    *   Willingness to listen
    *   Loving kindness
    *   Humor

4. Why might it be hard to approach *co-worker A* in a more spiritual way?
5. How would you identify with *co-worker B's* situation from your heart?
6. What questions might you ask *co-worker B* so you might understand her situation better?
7. What characteristics would you need if you were to approach *co-worker B* in a more spiritual way? Examples might include the following:
    *   Patience
    *   Willingness to listen
    *   Humor
    *   Loving kindness
    *   Understanding
    *   Gentleness

8. Would it be easier to approach *co-worker A* or *co-worker B* in a more spiritual way? Why?

Share with participants that when they put themselves in someone else's shoes, it can become easier to understand why the person behaved the way he or she did. It also can help them respond more appropriately instead of reacting and feeling stressed out. Share also with participants that they will have another opportunity to try to understand the importance of coping with stressful situations in a more spiritual way.

Note: Place all of the index cards that were filled out by the participants in a basket.

Have participants pick an index card and consider what questions they might need to ask the person to better understand what it could be like to "be in their co-worker's shoes?" How could they respond more spiritually? Invite them to share their responses with the group.

> "And if we observe humans who are two years old, we find that most of the time these humans have a big smile on their face and they are having fun. They are exploring the world. They are not afraid to play. They are afraid when they are hurt, when they are hungry, when some of their needs are not met, but they don't worry about the past, don't care about the future and only live in the present moment."
>
> —Don Miguel Ruiz, from *The Four Agreements*

CORE EXERCISE (35 minutes)
Missed Opportunities

Tools Needed
- Flip chart
- Markers
- Construction paper
- Handouts 7.2 , 7.3, 7.4, and 7.5

Tell participants that they will be engaging in a short discussion as a group on the differences are between having a soulful experience and having a stressful experience. Discuss Handout 7.2, asking participants to share some examples of both *soulful* and *stressful* experiences.

Share with participants that they will now have an opportunity to apply some of the concepts they just learned in a game format. The object of the game is to see if participants can figure out how each situation could be *an opportunity to respond in a more spiritual way*. Each time they answer correctly, they score a point. At the end of the game, the team with the most points wins.

Note: Handout 7.3 provides the various scenarios containing the missed opportunities and Handout 7.4 serves as the answer key for this exercise.

At the end of the game, give the participants Handout 7.5 on meditation. The trainer should read the explanation of what the meditation is and mention that participants can use this meditation when they are feeling stressed.

Ask participants to share why it is important to be able to identify opportunities and missed opportunities to cope with stress in a more spiritual way.

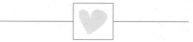

Closing (5 minutes)

 Thank participants for their willingness to participate in this training today and ask them to complete the evaluation form.

Evaluation Questions

1. Did you find this training helpful? (circle one)   Yes   No
   Please explain why or why not.

   _____
   _____
   _____
   _____

2. Will you be able to use the information
   you learned today at work? (circle one)   Yes   No

   _____
   _____
   _____
   _____

3. Do you believe this information will help you cope
   with stress differently? (circle one) Please explain.   Yes   No

   _____
   _____
   _____
   _____

4. What might be some ways to cope with stress from a more spiritual approach?
   Give at least two examples.

   _____
   _____
   _____
   _____

5. How did you feel after this workshop? (circle all that apply)

good	encouraged	cared about
sad	bored	listened to
frustrated	informed	angry
blessed	joyful	inspired
motivated	good about myself	

Being in Someone Else's Shoes

Co-worker A has not been feeling well. She has been very tired because her baby daughter has been cutting new teeth and has been keeping her from getting enough sleep for several days. She finds herself less patient and more easily angered than usual. She knows that she is taking her frustration out on co-worker B, but has not been able to do anything about it because she feels so stressed out. In the meantime, co-worker B has been very frustrated to the point of being angry with co-worker A, as she has not been pulling her load. Co-worker A also tends to make excuses and never apologizes for not doing her job. Co-worker B has had it; she feels stressed out and angry and finally yells at co-worker A. The two co-workers end up having a loud verbal argument in front of several residents.

How could this situation be handled in a more spiritual way?

If you were co-worker B, what questions could you ask co-worker A to better understand her situation?

If you were co-worker A, what questions could you ask co-worker B to better understand her situation?

Soulful Versus Stressful Experiences

Soulful Experience	Stressful Experience
Experience the moment	Worry about what might happen or has not happened
Come more from the heart, using intuition and feeling	Stay in the head, using judgment and ego
Appreciate all the abundance in your life	Focus on what you don't have and think about things in a negative way
Recognize the inner beauty of people and things; see a "crisis" as an *opportunity,* see a "failure" as a *learning experience*	Focus on what you don't like about a person; see a situation as a failure or terrible crisis
Love unconditionally	Love only because you want approval or seek to please someone
Be still and quiet	Stay busy and constantly doing something
Be open and willing to be flexible or to give up control	Believe things are to be done only your way and stay *task-centered* instead of *heart-centered*
Acknowledge and express anger appropriately	Hold in your anger until you explode or get sick
Be kind and gentle to yourself	Be hard on yourself and punish yourself by overeating, drinking alcohol, or participating in other harmful behaviors

Missed Opportunities

Instructions

Try to figure out what the *missed opportunities* and the *opportunities* are in each scenario. The trainer will read each scenario out loud.

Scenario One

You have to be at work at 7:00 a.m. You know it takes 45 minutes with traffic to get to work. You are always good about making sure you leave yourself plenty of time. Today you left a bit later than you normally do. As you head to work you remember that you have a meeting that will start right at 7:00 a.m. You drive faster than you should to make up for the late start. You are halfway to work when traffic comes to a standstill. You start to get frustrated and worried that you will never make it to work for the meeting. As you creep along, you continue to look at your watch and realize you will definitely be late. You start swearing at the traffic and then get upset with yourself. You start to think about excuses for why you are late. You arrive at work upset and stressed out. You walk into the meeting knowing your supervisor is going to be upset with you, so you make up an excuse to tell her. Just as you are about to tell your excuse she says, "I heard there was an awful accident and was so worried that you could have been hurt."

Scenario Two

You are driving home from work after a long and stressful day. You were working short staffed, and, for whatever reason, the residents were particularly challenging. You can't wait to get home. It starts to rain. Before long, traffic comes almost to a halt. "Darn, an accident," you think, "just my luck." You sit in traffic for about 10 minutes. The sun comes out and a beautiful rainbow appears. You notice the rainbow but still feel frustrated about being stuck in awful traffic.

Scenario Three

You are so mad at your best friend. She said something that was hurtful and uncaring. You are so hurt that you decide you don't ever want to talk with her. She calls you, and you don't return her calls. Months go by, and then you find out from another friend that her mother had a stroke and died.

Scenario Four

You come home from work and your spouse/partner starts talking with you. You are really not in the mood to listen, so you pretend to listen but you are really thinking about something completely different.

Scenario Five

You are talking with your supervisor about an issue concerning a resident. You have very strong feelings about how it should be handled. You are so determined that it should be resolved *your way* that you become very frustrated and angry and hear nothing that your boss is saying.

Scenario Six

You are in a hurry to get all your residents bathed before the end of your shift. You go to bathe Mr. X, but he wants to show you a medal he received a long time ago when he was in the army. You have seen that medal and need to get going. You tell him you can't look and hurry him into his bath. He gets a bit agitated and you end up having difficulty bathing him.

Missed Opportunities—Answer Key

Scenario One

Missed Opportunity

You could have taken some deep breaths to calm yourself so that when you got to work you would be able to say you were sorry for being late and not feel like you had to invent an excuse. You could have played soothing music or listened to a book on tape to distract yourself from the stress of having to be in horrible traffic. Because you worked yourself up and made a judgment about how your boss would respond, you risked *missing an opportunity* to experience your boss in a positive way.

Opportunity

You share with your boss that you are indeed sorry for being late, that you didn't give yourself enough time, and that you take responsibility for it. You prepare for stressful traffic so that when you run into it, you will not feel so upset about it.

Scenario Two

Missed Opportunity

You missed the opportunity to enjoy a beautiful rainbow, be in the moment, and allow yourself to experience a *gift* that the universe gave you.

Opportunity

You allow yourself to enjoy the rainbow and feel blessed that it was there to take the place of the awful traffic you are in.

Scenario Three

Missed Opportunity

By holding a grudge, you missed the opportunity of being there for a close friend's significant life event.

Opportunity

You could have given her the opportunity to explain why she said what she said and then made your decision about whether to remain friends.

Scenario Four

Missed Opportunity

You missed the opportunity to connect with your spouse/partner and share something of potential importance or significance because you were not present in the moment.

Opportunity

You could have had a connection with your spouse/partner that potentially could have been significant or important.

Scenario Five

Missed Opportunity

You missed the opportunity for considering another way of thinking about the issue and possibly even learning from the situation.

Opportunity

You could have been open to learning from your supervisor or found a way to share your opinion without making a judgment.

Scenario Six

Missed Opportunity

You miss learning something about Mr. X that might help you understand him better or help him feel *heard* and ultimately *cared about.* You also miss being able to be with him from your heart.

Opportunity

You get a chance to connect with Mr. X from a *heart place,* and you can feel good having listened to him.

Loving-Kindness Meditation

*"In this life we cannot do great things.
We can only do small things with great love."*
—Mother Teresa

The things in our life that matter the most are not "fantastic" or "grand." They are the *moments* when we touch one another, when we are there in the most attentive and caring way. These moments of touching and being touched can become a foundation for the path of the heart.

To love fully and live well requires us to recognize that we do not possess or own anything—our homes, our cars, our loved ones, not even our own bodies. Spiritual joy and wisdom do not come through possession but rather through our capacity to open, to love more fully (Kornfield, 1993).

What is Meditation?

Meditation is a way to connect to ourselves and to our hearts quietly, intentionally, and lovingly. The only thing you need to meditate is a place that is comfortable so that you can quiet the mind and connect to the heart. "The Loving-Kindness Meditation" was developed by Jack Kornfield, author of the book *A Path with Heart,* as a way to help people slow down, let go of the stress in their life, and realize the abundance and love in life.

When you sit down to try the meditation, make sure you can take the time to just *BE*—to be quiet with yourself and your surroundings, uninterrupted by children, grandchildren, spouses, neighbors, and so forth. Find a place to relax fully, whether in a favorite chair, in a garden, on a porch, or on a couch. Close your eyes and take deep breaths. Breathe in and then breathe out, listening to your breathing and being attentive to it. Listen also to your heartbeat. It is amazing what our bodies do every day that we pay little attention to and take for granted. Then, in your head or out loud, say the Loving-Kindness Meditation below.

If you attempt to try this meditation daily, it might give you an opportunity to get more in touch with what is truly important in your life. It surely will slow you down even for just a short while and let your body rest. What the meditation is attempting to do is help us *connect* in a loving way to the people in our lives with whom we come into contact every day. In addition, it is equally important to connect in a loving way to ourselves! As people who work in the helping fields, we too often ignore taking care of ourselves while we are busy taking care of others.

Loving-Kindness Meditation   *May I be filled with loving kindness*
May I be well
May I be peaceful and at ease
May I be happy

As you say this meditation, let the feelings arise with the words. Repeat the phrases over and over again, letting the feelings go all through your body and mind.

This is a meditation that can help each of us connect to our hearts and be aware of how to connect to others in a *heartful* way.

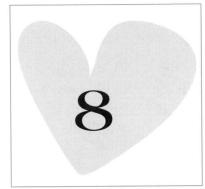

Communicating from the Heart

8

"The eyes believe themselves; the ears believe others;
and the heart believes the truth."
—Ibo, from *A Tiny Treasury of African Proverbs*

"It is better in prayer to have a heart without
words than words without a heart."
—Mahatma Gandhi

OBJECTIVES

- To teach ways to encourage a spiritual approach to communication

- To help leadership recognize the barriers to effective communication

- To provide effective communication tools

WHAT IT MEANS TO COMMUNICATE FROM THE HEART

In her book *Kitchen Table Wisdom,* author Rachel Naomi Remen says the following about communication:

> I suspect that the most basic and powerful way to connect to another person is to listen. Just listen. Perhaps the most important thing we ever give each other is our attention. And especially if it's given from the heart. When people are talking, there's no need to do anything but receive them. Just take them in. Listen to what they're saying. Care about it. Most times caring about it is even more important than under-

standing it…

…Listening is the oldest and perhaps the most powerful tool of healing. It is often through the quality of our listening and not the wisdom of our words that we are able to effect the most profound changes on the people around us. When we listen, we offer with our attention an opportunity for wholeness.

When we communicate from the heart, we listen to people's souls. A loving silence has far more power to heal and to connect than the most well-intentioned words. When we really listen with our hearts and put our minds aside, we hear and see with commitment and caring.

When leadership communicates in this way, the communication takes on special meaning. It models for everyone being able to hear the heart and see the soul. It promotes authentic communication.

In working with elders, the importance of listening from the heart cannot be underestimated; the thoughts of Rachel Naomi Remen regarding the significance that listening holds for communication are particularly important. As staff members work with the physical, emotional, and cognitive challenges facing elders—including sensory impairments, chronic illnesses, dementia, and depression—they find that listening from the heart becomes even more critical to effective communication. Although the culturally accepted way to communicate is through words, for example, this traditional communication channel is often not effective or available to elders with Alzheimer's disease or dementia who may have lost their ability to speak or use words. Therefore, staff members have to learn to be comfortable with other modes of communication. They will find that they have to listen more intently and show that they are doing so through touching, smiling, and sitting close to the elder. In addition, they have to pay close attention to the way the elder is communicating by observing the elder's nonverbal behavior and facial expressions. The most important thing to remember when communicating with an elder who has language or cognitive challenges is to convey to that elder that you care and will listen.

If an elder is depressed or experiencing a loss, finding a way just to listen and show that you care is what matters most. Professionals do not need to take away what elders are feeling or try to fix it. Sometimes sitting with someone in a loving, caring connection and just listening to him or her is the best way to be. Giving the elder your full attention is a gift of listening from the heart. It is far more effective than words can ever be.

"Silence provides time for our souls to be present.
We are used to being present in our heads,
our minds, our intellects."
—Kay Lindahl, from *The Sacred Art of Listening*

THE ART OF LISTENING

In our culture, we are not really taught how to listen. We might remember echoes of our parents' stern voices saying to us, "Be quiet, just listen!" or "Listen to what I am telling you!" The messages we received as young children conveyed that listening was something you had to do when you were bad or if you were not agreeing with what was being told to you. Thus, to some extent, we receive either negative or at least mixed messages about listening.

We are not formally trained to listen. There are no courses in elementary or high school to teach basic listening skills. In college, the only way students learn the skills of listening is if they take a human services course, which typically offers skills in listening, interviewing techniques, or crisis intervention.

In today's world, there is little room for listening. We are always in a hurry or concerned with multi-tasking. How many of us are truly listening when we chat on the phone with a friend while surfing the Internet or cooking dinner? When our spouse or partner comes home from work and starts talking to us, how often do we pretend to listen when, in fact, we are thinking about what we need to do next? Every day we are exposed to poor listening at work, at home, on television, and in movies and plays; people are constantly interrupting each other, yelling to get their point across, and talking over one another.

The truth, however, is that listening transcends our beliefs and words. It transcends gender, socioeconomic status, culture, and age. If we listen authentically, then we listen with our whole being—mind, body, and spirit. In working with elders and listening from the whole of one's self, a ripple effect begins in how the elders respond and how the professionals respond. The elders feel cared about and valued, and staff members feel good that they feel good! When a facility's leadership and staff listen authentically, they are giving the gift of caring.

Listening is a skill everyone can learn, but it does take practice. It requires making choices—either to listen or not to listen. And if we choose to listen, we need to listen with intention, commitment, and awareness. We must be fully present. Certain skills can help to develop a deeper level of listening and communicating, which I define as *spiritual listening* and describe in Module 8, which follows. Training Module 8 was developed to help participants recognize the different ways to communicate from the heart that can lead them to find the gifts in listening.

REFERENCES

Remen, R.N. (1996). *Kitchen table wisdom: Stories that heal.* New York: Riverhead Books.

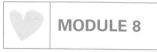 **MODULE 8** | # Communicating from the Heart

INTRODUCTION (10 minutes)

> **Tools Needed**
> - Flip chart
> - Markers

 Have participants introduce themselves. Ask them to share a situation in which they were trying to communicate something and it backfired on them or was completely misunderstood.

Share with participants what they should expect to learn from this module and list these expectations on the flip chart.
- Participants will have a clearer understanding of how to communicate more compassionately and from the heart.
- Participants will be able to define *spiritual listening*.
- Participants will learn new skills for authentic listening.
- Participants will be able to identify ways that listening can connect them to one another and to the elders with whom they work.

 Ask participants if there are other expectations they would like to include and write these on the flip chart.

WARM-UP EXERCISE (30 minutes)
The Balloon

> **Tools Needed**
> - Flip chart
> - Markers

 Explain to participants that they are going to participate in an exercise that demonstrates the power of communication without words.

Note: You are going to pantomime blowing up a balloon by pretending to reach into your pocket and pull out a balloon. Stretch the balloon as you prepare to blow it up, then blow deep breaths into the balloon three or four times until it has expanded. You can indicate with your hands that the balloon is getting bigger and bigger until it finally needs to be tied up.

Explain to participants that they are to line up one behind the other, standing front to back. When it is their turn, they are to pay close attention to what is pantomimed to them. Start with the first person in the line and communicate the pantomime. After that person receives the pantomime, he or she will then tap the person behind him or her and repeat the pantomime to that person, trying to remember all the details of the pantomime. It should proceed down the line until it reaches the last person. When the final person receives the pantomime, he or she is to pantomime it to the whole group.

Note: Usually by the time it reaches the last person, the pantomime is completely different. The trainer should not share how the pantomime has changed with the group until it is finished.

Have participants share some examples of the barriers to communication that resulted from this exercise. Write their responses on the flip chart. Be sure to share the following points about *listening:*

- It involves our whole being. It is not only listening for words but also paying attention to the mind, body, and spirit of communication, as demonstrated in the exercise. Often people say much more to us than just the words they use.
- It increases awareness of how communication can be *interpreted* differently.
- It demonstrates how all people have their *own perspective* on the way they see things.
- It demonstrates the importance of "checking out" what has been communicated to make sure it has been received as it was intended.
- It increases awareness of how *paying attention* is not enough and that *understanding* is also needed.
- It demonstrates the power of nonverbal communication.

"When the eyes see what they have never seen before,
the heart feels what it has never felt."
—Balthasar Gracian

CORE EXERCISE (50 minutes)
Finding the Gifts in Listening

> **Tools needed**
> - Flip chart
> - Markers
> - Handouts 8.1, 8.2, 8.3, and 8.4

Explain to participants that there are many different ways to listen. *The Caring Spirit* approach emphasizes spiritual listening—a process by which the listener intentionally prepares him- or herself for listening compassionately and from the heart. It requires a deeper level of listening, because the listener is making a choice to listen authentically. Listening authentically means listening with compassion, honesty, and caring, and without judgment.

Note: Have the participants refer to Handouts 8.1 and 8.2 for an in-depth discussion of spiritual listening and the possible roadblocks to communication.

The following skills are involved in spiritual listening:
- The ability of the listener to be able to quiet his or her mind. The quieting of the mind makes room for the listener to absorb with full attention what is being said to him or her.
- The willingness of the listener to remain compassionate, even when what is said triggers uncomfortable emotions.
- The ability to be patient. When people are in a hurry, they tend to only half listen or to rush the person who is communicating with them. Being patient requires the listener to make a commitment to want to hear what is being communicated.
- The willingness to stay present and in the moment. With professionals' lives offering so much distraction, it is not easy to stay focused and present. This skill involves maintaining awareness and an open mind, and having an environment that is free from distraction.
- The ability to be honest in listening, which involves letting the person know when the listener is unable to give full attention to what is being shared. If professionals are distracted, preoccupied, or tired and unable to focus, they are only half listening.
- The ability to be comfortable with silence and still stay connected to the person. As Kay Lindahl points out in her book *Practicing the Sacred Art of Listening,* the letters in the word LISTEN also spell SILENT. Being able to connect in silence with someone is an important communication skill that is not always easy to do.
- The ability to recognize listening as sacred. When professionals can see listening as a gift, it changes the way listening is valued. It encourages a mutual experience for both the listener and communicator. In addition, it provides both individuals with the opportunity for positive connection.

Explain to participants that spiritual listening takes practice. Participants will now have the opportunity to practice some of the skills needed to be a spiritual listener. Participants will break into small groups. Each group will be given a scenario that will require them to practice the skills needed to be more effective spiritual listeners. Identify which scenario in Handout 8.3 each group will explore. After they have practiced these skills, they will have the opportunity to share their scenarios with the whole group.

Note: Provide Handout 8.4 for the discussion of the scenarios by the whole group.

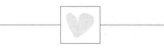

Closing (5 minutes)

The trainer should summarize for the participants the following main concepts of spiritual listening:
- Being compassionate
- Listening for understanding because you care
- Listening patiently, instead of hurrying the person
- Being fully present
- Listening honestly
- Talking *to* the person, not *over* the person as if he or she cannot understand or is not there
- Being intentional; making the choice to listen with full attention
- Recognizing listening as sacred
- Recognizing the gifts in listening

Mention that you hope participants have a better understanding of the importance of communicating from the heart.

Ask participants to fill out the evaluation form.

Evaluation Questions

1. Did you find this training helpful? (circle one)   Yes   No
   Please explain why or why not.

   _____

   _____

   _____

   _____

2. Will you be able to use the information
   you learned today at work? (circle one)   Yes   No
   Please list at least two examples.

   _____

   _____

   _____

   _____

3. What are some of the *barriers* to communicating with people?
   List at least two examples.

   _____

   _____

   _____

   _____

4. How might you communicate in a more spiritual way? List a few examples.

   _____

   _____

   _____

   _____

5. How did you feel after this workshop? (circle all that apply)

good	encouraged	cared about
sad	bored	listened to
frustrated	informed	angry
blessed	joyful	inspired
motivated	good about myself	

Spiritual Listening

"Listening is the oldest and perhaps the most powerful tool of healing. It is often through the quality of our listening and not the wisdom of our words that we are able to effect the most profound changes on the people around us."
—Rachel Naomi Remen, from *Kitchen Table Wisdom*

Spiritual listening is a process by which you, the listener, intentionally prepare yourself for listening compassionately and from the heart. It requires a deeper level of listening because you are making a choice to listen authentically. There are particular skills involved in spiritual listening:

- You must be able to quiet your mind. The quieting of the mind makes room for absorbing with full attention what is being said to you.
- You must be willing to remain compassionate even when what is being communicated triggers uncomfortable emotions.
- You must be patient. We are often in a hurry and tend only to half listen to or rush the person who is communicating with us. Being patient requires you to make a commitment to hear what is being communicated.
- You must be willing to stay present and in the moment. Our lives contain so much distraction, it is not easy to stay focused and present. This skill involves consciously maintaining an open mind and making sure the environment we are communicating in is free from distraction.
- You must be honest in your listening and let the person know when you are not able to listen or give your full attention. If we are distracted, preoccupied, or tired and unable to focus, then our thoughts get in the way and we are only half listening.
- You need to be comfortable with silence and still be able to stay connected to the person. As author Kay Lindahl points out in her book *Practicing the Sacred Art of Listening,* the letters in the word LISTEN also spell SILENT. Being able to connect in silence with someone is an important communication skill that is not always easy to do.
- You must be able to find the gifts in listening and to view listening as sacred. When we can see listening as a *gift,* it changes the way we value it. A mutual experience develops for both the listener and the communicator. Both individuals have the opportunity for positive connection.

Communication Roadblocks

Being aware of the obstacles to communication can help you communicate more clearly and with less misunderstanding. The following are the most common *road-blocks* to effective communication:

- **Willingness to listen:** How open are the receiver and sender to *really listening* and not judging?
- **Emotional state:** What is the emotional state of the sender or receiver, such as stressed, depressed, anxious, angry, happy, excited, playful, or tired?
- **Attitude:** Is the sender sending a positive or negative message, and how open is the receiver?
- **Perception:** Is the message or information expressed being perceived in a way that is different than it was intended?
- **Relationship of the communicators:** Do the people communicating care about each other or care about how the information is received?
- **Distraction:** Is the environment appropriate for sending and receiving the information?
- **Intention/meaning:** Is the message or information carefully considered or said quickly and without much thought?
- **Context:** Is the information being delivered for the right situation?
- **Sensory impairments:** Does either the sender or receiver have sensory deficits that make hearing or understanding the information difficult?

Spiritual Listening Exercise

Scenario One

Mrs. Jones is 85 years old. She has been widowed for 2 years. She had been living in Cleveland, Ohio, and for a while managed to take care of herself despite having Parkinson's disease. However, as her Parkinson's disease became worse, everyday tasks became more difficult. Her adult children were worried and decided she needed to move out of the home she had lived in for 40 years to live nearer to them. At the time, she agreed.

Mrs. Jones moved into an assisted living facility closer to her children, who live in Georgia. Since moving and selling her home, she has become angry. She is taking her anger and sadness out on the caregivers who work with her. She is curt with the caregivers and sometimes refuses to let them help her, even though she does need help with ADLs. She is cognitively intact, but appears to be depressed.

As Mrs. Jones' caregiver, how would you utilize your spiritual listening skills in caring for her?

Questions to Consider

1. Are you able to quiet your mind and listen with an open heart?
2. Can you find a way to be compassionate and not judge?
3. Do you care enough to want to listen?
4. Can you find the gifts in listening to Mrs. Jones despite how she is communicating?

Scenario Two

Mr. Johns is a 79-year-old who lives in his own home. He was never married and concentrated his life on his work. He is a retired general. He traveled all over the world and is very proud of his accomplishments. He does not have dementia but tends to tell the same stories over and over again. You are his caregiver and you find his stories boring. You listen anyway because you don't want to hurt his feelings.

Questions to Consider

1. Are you listening because you want to understand Mr. Johns or because you care about what is being communicated?
2. Are you listening with full attention and really hearing what he is saying or are you half listening?
3. Are you keeping an open mind?
4. Are you quieting your own mind so you can take in what he is sharing, or are you thinking about something else because you are bored with the same stories?

Scenario Three

You work for a home care agency and are taking care of a 93-year-old woman named Mrs. Kaiser. Lately your personal life has been very stressful. Your son has been sick, your husband has been working extra hours, and you feel like everything is on your shoulders. You go to work tired and stressed out. Sometimes it seems like your day will never end. Plus, Mrs. Kaiser has cognitive challenges and does not understand what you say to her most of the time. You feel like you just want to throw your hands up and quit!

Questions to Consider

1. How can you find a way to be patient?
2. Can you stay focused in the present moment so your personal life doesn't intrude?

Scenario Four

You work in a nursing home and are responsible for 10 residents every day you come to work. You find there is hardly enough time in the day just to do the work you need to do. The other caregiver who works on your hall has been continually talking to you about her personal life. You half listen to her and try to hurry her along because you have to take care of your residents. You really don't want to hurt her feelings, but you don't have the time to spend with her and also do your job.

Questions to Consider

1. When should you let a person know you are not fully listening?
2. Do you need to be more patient and compassionate?

Spiritual Listening Answers

Scenario One Answers

When an elder is treating caregivers poorly or talking to them in an angry, curt manner, it is easy to take it personally and become defensive. It becomes difficult to keep your heart open and to stay compassionate.

If you were the caregiver working with Mrs. Jones and were to apply the skills of spiritual listening, you would want to do the following:

- Move beyond her words and get to the underlying emotions: her pain and sadness. It is not always easy to do this, but when you can, the rewards are well worth the effort. Letting her know you hear her pain and sadness helps her to feel that she is being heard, that she matters, and that you care.
- You can't fix her or her feelings, but you can listen with full attention.
- Just listening provides a gift to her of having the opportunity to express her feelings and be heard. Plus, it gives you the opportunity to practice patience, compassion, and staying connected to your heart.

Scenario Two Answers

This is a common situation, feeling you *have* to listen to the person to avoid being rude. Sometimes we even believe we must listen so we don't hurt the person's feelings.

If you were the caregiver for Mr. Johns and applied the skills of spiritual listening in this situation you would need to find a way to hear Mr. Johns' stories from a different perspective. You might want to consider the following:

- Learn to shift how you listen by concentrating less on the *content* of the story and more on the *feelings* behind the story. This approach helps you listen in a deeper way. You could also shift the content by asking him questions about the story that would be more interesting to you, offering an opportunity for mutual connection.
- Recognize how proud Mr. Johns feels about his accomplishments and tell him so, which validates for him that you care. This is the gift you give him by your listening.
- Understand how being patient and making the commitment to listening offers a way to listen to him with a different ear.
- What does it mean to give your full attention? If you are tired or are thinking about something else, then you need to let him know you are unable to listen fully. It is important to stop him before he gets too involved with his storytelling. You might say something like the following: "Mr. Johns, you have some great stories, and I know how much they mean to you, but I can't give you my full attention now." If he still wants to tell his story, you need to let him know that you are not fully listening.

Scenario Three Answers

To apply the skills of spiritual listening with Mrs. Kaiser, you would need to consider the following:

- Try staying present and in the moment. You would have to learn to put your own life stresses aside so that you could tune into and be present to Mrs. Kaiser. This means learning how to draw on those resources that give you strength and courage.
- Find other ways to communicate with Mrs. Kaiser besides just using words. Maybe holding her hand, smiling, singing, dancing, or praying could be ways that would let her know you are listening to her. Plus, those ways of communicating can be mutually satisfying for both of you.

Scenario Four Answers

If you were the caregiver in this situation and applied the spiritual listening skills needed to work through this problem, you might consider the following:

- Be willing to be patient. Patience is the key to making the commitment and wanting to listen to what is bothering your co-worker.
- Let her know when you are not able to listen fully because you are distracted by your work. You might suggest that you both find a time that would be mutually agreeable when you could listen more freely to her.

The Caring Spirit Approach to Eldercare: A Training Guide for Professionals and Families
by Nancy L. Kriseman © 2005 Health Professions Press, Inc. All rights reserved.

Staying Connected Through Rituals

"Our lives are an endless ritual."
—Robert Fulghum, from *From Beginning to End*

OBJECTIVES

- To help leadership understand why the concept of ritual is important for staff members and those for whom they care

- To be able to define the different types of rituals present in western culture

- To highlight how rituals can connect staff and elders

- To sensitize leadership and staff to the importance of respecting and valuing cultural difference and diversity among themselves and the elders with whom they work

DEFINITION OF RITUALS

Every culture in the world has created rituals to guide and ease people through life's passages. Rituals connect people to their families, friends, and communities and connect the past to the present. Rituals offer us opportunities to explore the meaning of life in the following ways:

- They provide anchors and markers that make life's passages visible.

- They are reminders of the shifts and transitions in life, and they often provide support throughout these passages.

119

- They provide ways to honor and celebrate life individually, with families, and in community.

Rituals are intertwined in all areas of our lives in the following ways:

- They arise from the stages and ages of life.

- They transform the ordinary into the holy or extraordinary.

- They can be public, private, or completely secret.

- They are in constant evolution and transformation.

- They reflect and create the values of a culture.

There are many rituals in everyone's life that hold particular meaning and that are important to the quality of life. Without these rituals, many people would feel lost or depressed; life would hold less meaning.

When I reflect on the rituals of my childhood, I become somewhat sad. I miss some of those rituals, especially the ones that involved my family and friends. I smile when I think about the Saturday ritual I had with my dad of going downtown and eating foot-long hot dogs with everything on them. It was such a special treat and something I looked forward to doing with him. I am currently a vegetarian, but I can still taste, smell, and remember the wonderful times dad and I had together. Or when mom and I would watch Lucille Ball each week, laughing hysterically while filling ourselves with potato chips and sour cream. I can also remember how all my friends and I would gather every day after school in my basement and pretend we were the Beatles. We would sing their songs and put on performances for the neighborhood. This kept us occupied for hours and was a ritual we engaged in for years. As simple, and even silly, as some of my childhood rituals were, they were an important part of my childhood. I recognize how these rituals kept me grounded, supported me through some difficult times, and helped me feel like I belonged.

UNDERSTANDING RITUALS

In their book *Rituals of Our Times,* authors Evan Imber-Black and Janine Roberts suggested that rituals are a central part of life, whether through the sharing of meals or major life-cycle events. By practicing rituals, the emotional connections to parents, spouses/partners, children, siblings, and dear friends can be strengthened and maintained. The authors added that rituals provide a path to the future when ceremonies, traditions, objects, symbols, and ways of being with each other are passed down through generations.

Imber-Black and Roberts related that all rituals contain symbols and symbolic actions. These are generally unique to a particular culture, family, couple, or individual. They can also contain religious meaning.

Symbols often express far more than words. Often, a single object can create and express many different meanings. "Symbols give voice to our beliefs, inner feelings, relationships and spirituality," stated Imber-Black and Roberts. Symbols are included in our daily rituals, traditions, holiday celebrations, and life-cycle passages. Examples of symbols might include the following:

- Cakes
- Clothes
- Special foods
- Presents
- Flowers

Symbolic actions are the way symbols are carried out. Symbolic actions are actions and behaviors that imbue rituals with meaning. Symbolic actions help express behavior in either cultural or religious rituals, many of which may be hundreds of years old. Symbolic actions are also found in our daily rituals and life-cycle passages. Examples of symbolic actions might include the following:

- Throwing caps in the air in a graduation ceremony

- Placing flowers on a grave in honor of Father's or Mother's Day

- Exchanging wedding vows and rings

- Blowing the *schofar* (ram's horn) during the Jewish high holidays

- Easter egg hunts in celebration of Easter

- Taking communion

FOUR TYPES OF RITUALS

Imber-Black and Roberts identified the following four major types of rituals:

- Daily rituals

- Holidays

- Traditions

- Life-cycle passages

Daily Rituals

The large and small rituals that fill our daily lives arise from a range of needs and serve various functions. Because of their diversity, these rituals can be grouped by what motivates us to do them.

Meaningful Rituals

Meaningful rituals are something one values doing each day and wants to make time for. Examples of these might include:

- Exercising every morning or evening

- Meditating each day

- Showering in the morning or evening
- Calling one's parent to see how he or she is doing
- Reading a bedtime story to one's son or daughter

Obligatory Daily Rituals

Obligatory rituals are those that people feel must be done each day, even if they are not enjoyable or meaningful. They might include:

- Exercising even though the person actually dislikes it
- Talking on the telephone to a parent out of duty, not pleasure
- Going to work at a job one really does not like
- Reading the paper to stay current with the news

Rigid Rituals

In more limited circumstances there are rituals that are *rigid* in nature. These might be rituals that have little room for flexibility and might include the following:

- Carpooling kids to school
- Having to be at work at a certain time
- Eating lunch at a certain time
- Taking a medication at a certain time

Voluntary Rituals

Some rituals are more voluntary in nature. These rituals often include choices as to when and how they are done and might include:

- Volunteering for a job
- Choosing to carpool or take the bus to work
- Making lunch for a spouse/partner

What appears to be most important about one's daily rituals is being aware of how they affect one's life and whether they are meaningful to that individual.

Traditions, Holidays, and Life-Cycle Passages

Imber-Black and Roberts have an interesting way of categorizing rituals of *life-cycle passages* and *holidays* and/or *traditions*. They described them as rituals that are "inside and outside the calendar," respectively. They defined "outside the calendar" rituals as rituals that are not *marked* or *celebrated* on the calendar our society observes. These rituals can be joyous or sad and give a great deal of meaning to life. They also can be voluntary. These "outside the calendar" rituals are typically more flexible and tend to be more personal. Examples include:

• Anniversaries	• Vacations	• Birthdays	• Reunions
• Deaths	• Divorces	• Weddings	

• Certain religious celebrations: christenings, baby namings, bar/bat mitzvahs, confirmations

"Inside the calendar" rituals are defined as holidays and/or traditions that are *marked* on society's calendars as events that will always take place on those particular dates. They tend to be more rigid and can even have obligatory features to them. Examples might include:

• Holidays such as Martin Luther King Jr. Day, Christmas, Rosh Hashanah, Memorial Day, Mother's Day, and Independence Day

• Events such as baseball's World Series and football's Super Bowl that taake place in a fixed and expected season

How one participates in a ritual will often depend on whether the ritual is seen as meaningful, voluntary, rigid, or obligatory.

On a personal note, as I grow older I find ritual does not have to involve words, occasions, or celebrations to be meaningful. I am trying to create a ritual of learning to find sacred time for silence in my life on a regular basis, whether it is intentional, such as meditation or emptying my mind before I go to sleep at night, or not. The ritual of silence is powerful and too often neglected. Yet, some of the most powerful rituals are those that are reflective or that invoke silence. For example, I think about the ritual of sitting in front of my fireplace every winter and how wonderful that feels. During springtime, I sit in my garden each day before I go to work, watching the birds and taking in the smells and beauty that is all around me.

THE IMPORTANCE OF RITUAL IN ELDERS' LIVES

"The rituals are cairns marking the path behind us and ahead of us. Without them we lose our way."
—Robert Fulghum, from *From Beginning to End*

Celebrating and honoring rituals are ways to help elders stay connected to their faith community and are a way of validating and respecting their cultural heritage. Encouraging ritual in the lives of elders can also influence how they feel about themselves. When they have the opportunity to celebrate or practice a ritual that is meaningful to them, it reinforces feelings of comfort and of feeling valued, cared about, and respected.

Gerontologists and other health professionals acknowledge the central role of rituals in the lives of elders (Imber-Black & Roberts, 1992; Koenig, 1999). The literature abounds with examples of how cultural heritage and ritual provide elders with

- A sense of pride about their history and background

- Validation that they have been through difficult times and survived those times

- Friendships among their religious or cultural heritage community, which engender common background and help to encourage a sense of trust and intimacy

- Strong ties and powerful connections to their family

- A sense of belonging and security

- Linkage to their past and to the present

Rituals and traditions, such as prayers, are an enduring aspect of self-identity for older adults. In my work with elders, I have found this to be even truer with elders who have dementia. Although their ability to recall and remember recent events is limited or not present at all, they often recall the music or prayers of their religious or childhood backgrounds with ease.

The need for rituals and traditions is heightened among elders who have dementia, according to Virginia Bell and David Troxel, authors of several articles and books on dementia and spirituality. Therefore, finding ways to teach staff members how to encourage the religious, spiritual, and ritualistic aspects of the elders with whom they work is paramount to good care. Helping staff members learn ways to bring forth the life stories, cultural beliefs, and rituals of those in their care will demonstrate to staff members how they create meaning in the lives of those elders.

STORIES INVOLVING RITUALS

Rituals are very important in my therapy sessions with clients, and I often see elders in nursing homes brighten when they are involved in religious or cultural celebrations. For example, when I was a social worker in a Presbyterian nursing home in Atlanta, I conducted a group every month that focused on favorite religious or spiritual rituals of the residents. When it was my turn to pick a ritual or holiday to celebrate, I chose to celebrate Chanukah; it has always been one of my favorite holidays because of the meaning behind it and the wonderful ritual foods. I gathered my usual group of residents together and began to talk about Chanukah. I then started to make the potato pancakes (or *latkes*) that smell so good and taste delicious. I noticed that one of the men in my group was crying. I wheeled him away from the group and asked him why he was crying? He said that he was brought up Jewish, but then married a Presbyterian woman. All his married life he worshipped the Presbyterian faith because his wife said he could not marry her if he did not do so. My talking about Chanukah and cooking the ritual foods had brought back many memories for him. He sadly spoke of how he had missed practicing and participating in some of the Jewish rituals and holidays. I asked if he would like to begin again. He said yes, and fortunately I was able to arrange for a Rabbi and a student to visit him for all the Jewish holidays. After several visits from the Rabbi and student, I asked how he was enjoying them. He said, "I have gotten back a part of my identity and now I have a way to find meaning in my life since my wife died."

Another touching story is about a Jewish woman who was in the middle stages of Alzheimer's disease. She was living in an assisted living facility that was mostly Christian. Because I was a consultant in this facility, I had been conducting Passover Seders for the residents as a way of embracing different religious cultures. This particular woman was generally very quiet and had a difficult time expressing herself. She also had a tendency to wander. It was usually difficult to keep her focused on an activity. I decided to invite her to the Seder, not knowing what she would remember or if she would sit still long enough to participate. Much to everyone's surprise, she not only sat through the entire Seder, but she ate every morsel of food and participated in all the prayers and songs that I shared. The activities director was astounded. When I shared this story with the woman's daughter, she decided to pay special attention to the Jewish holidays and to make sure she celebrated them with her mother.

Training Module 9 was developed to help participants appreciate the importance of rituals in fostering spiritual relationships with elders.

REFERENCES

Bell, V., & Troxel, D. (2001). *Best Friends staff: Building a culture of care in Alzheimer's programs.* Baltimore: Health Professions Press.

Imber-Black, E., & Roberts, J. (1992). *Rituals for our times: Celebrating, healing, and changing our lives and our relationships.* New York: HarperCollins

Koenig, H.G. (1999). *The healing power of faith.* New York: Simon & Schuster.

	MODULE 9	# Staying Connected Through Rituals

"Public ceremonies crystallize personal
commitments, binding people together
and letting them know they are not alone."
—James Kouzes and Barry Posner, from *Encouraging the Heart*

INTRODUCTION (10 minutes)

Tools Needed
- Flip chart
- Markers

ask

Have participants introduce themselves. Ask them to share one family ritual that has been passed down from generation to generation. If they don't have a particular ritual, have them share one ritual they have created in their own family.

explain

Explain to participants what they should expect to learn from this module, and list these expectations on the flip chart.
- Participants will be able to understand how rituals connect them to themselves, their past, and their culture.
- Participants will be able to identify how rituals serve as markers and anchors in both their work and personal lives.
- Participants will be able to recognize the different types of rituals and how the rituals affect their lives.
- Participants will learn about the role that rituals play in the lives of elders for whom they care.

ask

Ask participants if there are other expectations they would like to include and write those on the flip chart.

WARM-UP EXERCISE (60 minutes)
It's All in the Ritual

> Tools Needed
> - Paper and pens
> - Handouts 9.1 and 9.2

Note: Share with participants some of the information in the chapter about the different types of rituals. Distribute Handout 9.1 and have participants read the description of rituals it presents.

 Explain to participants that they are to write down all the daily rituals they can think of from their personal lives. Encourage them to write down at least four or five examples. Then ask them to put a star next to the rituals that are the most meaningful to them. For example, participants might put a star next to one of the following rituals:
- Exercise daily
- Read a bedtime story to their child each night
- Kiss their spouse or partner goodbye, or at least say goodbye, before leaving for work
- Take a shower in the morning to help start their day

 Have participants share some of their most meaningful rituals with the group. Then explain to them that they can only keep one ritual that they wrote on their papers. Ask participants the following questions:
- What would your life be like if you had to let go of most of the daily rituals that were meaningful to you?
- What was the most difficult aspect of this exercise?
- How difficult do you think it is for the elders for whom you care to have to let go of their rituals? How might those elders feel?

> "The celebration aspect of rituals honors life
> with all its dilemmas, problems and difficulties.
> And with all its joys, successes and accomplishments.
> Sometimes just persevering in the face
> of enormous odds deserves a celebration."
> —Imber-Black and Roberts, from *Rituals for Our Times*

 Explain to participants that the next exercise will help them think of ways to mutually share rituals with the elders with whom they work. The trainer might want to help them explore the following questions as a way to help participants think of ideas:
- What is the cultural background of the elders in their care?
- What particular customs or traditions had been and still are important to the elder?

- What rituals seem most important for the elder to still practice?
- How can staff share their own cultural backgrounds and rituals without imposing them on the elders for whom they care?

 Share with participants that they will work in small groups and discuss each of the questions in Handout 9.2. They will have 10 minutes to discuss these questions and the ideas they have.

 Ask the participants to share their ideas with the group. The trainer might suggest the following ideas after participants have a chance to present their ideas:

- Recite daily prayers that are nonsectarian and that residents and staff could share together
- Sing or listen to music together
- Enjoy foods that staff members could either cook or bring in from each others' cultures and families
- Share pictures of the countries from which staff members and elders were born
- Sing lullabies or read stories that each group may have shared with their children
- Practice the dances that were popular in their culture
- Examine clothing and costumes specific to staff members' cultures
- Read poetry
- Engage in celebrations and holiday traditions

CORE EXERCISE (25 minutes)
Tour of Homes

Tools Needed
- Paper
- Pens

Note: Prior to this training session, the director of nursing or social worker will need to have requested permission from several residents to allow staff members to *tour* their personal space.

 Explain to participants that this exercise is designed to help them *see* and *experience* the elders with whom they work in a different way. One way to get to know the elders for whom they care in a more intimate way is to recognize their homes as places of "living history." Elders are the keepers of rituals in the form of memorabilia such as recipes, photo albums, special mementos, and other family treasures. They also are the carriers of ethnic heritage, as they hold knowledge of particular foods, songs, dances, and other rituals specific to their culture or ethnic group.

 Share with participants that they will have the opportunity to learn about the elders for whom they care by *touring* their homes. They will have about 10 minutes to tour the home and write down what they find and learn. Touring an elder's home means paying attention to the following things:
- *Symbols* that visibly show the elder's cultural heritage and religious background
- Ritual objects
- Objects or pictures that might have religious, cultural, or spiritual significance

 Gather participants together again and have them share what they found out about each elder. The trainer might ask them additional questions, such as:
- How might this information affect the way they care for elders?
- How did this information change their perception of that particular elder?
- Did they learn any information that might help them connect to one another, such as recognizing some commonalties spiritually, culturally, or religiously?

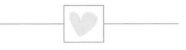

CLOSING (5 minutes)

 Thank the participants for their willingness to participate in the training. Mention that you hope they have a better understanding of how rituals affect everyone's lives.

Have participants fill out evaluations.

Evaluation Questions

1. Did you find this training helpful? (circle one)   Yes   No
    Please explain why or why not.

    _____

    _____

    _____

2. Will you be able to use the information
    you learned today at work? (circle one)   Yes   No
    If yes, give at least two examples.

    _____

    _____

    _____

3. Do you believe that learning about rituals will help you to
    care better for the elders in your care? (circle one)   Yes   No
    List at least two ways.

    _____

    _____

    _____

4. How could understanding an elder's cultural background
    help you in caring for him or her? List a few examples.

    _____

    _____

    _____

5. What might be some ways to share your cultural background
    and rituals with the elders with whom you work?

    _____

    _____

    _____

6. How did you feel after this workshop? (circle all that apply)

    good   encouraged   cared about
    sad   bored   listened to
    frustrated   informed   angry
    blessed   joyful   inspired
    motivated   good about myself

Rituals

"Our lives are an endless ritual."
—Robert Fulghum, from *From Beginning to End*

Rituals are important because

- They provide anchors and markers that make the visible known.
- They are reminders of the shifts and transitions in our lives and they provide support throughout those passages.
- They provide ways to honor and celebrate life individually, with families, and in community.
- They arise in all stages of our lives.
- They can be public, private, or secret.
- They are constantly changing.
- They reflect the values of our culture.

Rituals that are important to me

1. _____

2. _____

3. _____

4. _____

5. _____

6. _____

7. _____

8. _____

9. _____

10. _____

Questions to Ponder: Valuing Rituals

1. What is the cultural background of the elders you are caring for?

    _____
    _____
    _____
    _____
    _____
    _____

2. What particular customs or traditions had they
    celebrated and might still be interested in celebrating?

    _____
    _____
    _____
    _____
    _____
    _____

3. What rituals seem most important for the
    elders in your care to continue practicing?

    _____
    _____
    _____
    _____
    _____
    _____

4. How can you share your own traditions and background
    without imposing them on the elders with whom you work?

    _____
    _____
    _____
    _____
    _____
    _____

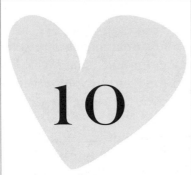

Taking Care of Our Own Spirits

10

"Those who have no compassion for themselves
have none for others either."
—Rabbi Meir

"I have only two remedies for weariness:
one is change and the other is relaxation."
—Eleanor Roosevelt, from *You Learn by Living*

OBJECTIVES

- To demonstrate the importance of teaching self-care skills to all staff who work in long-term care

- To help leadership define self-care in the workplace

- To teach leadership and the staff some spiritual tools that can help them take better care of themselves

UNDERSTANDING THE IMPORTANCE OF SELF-CARE FOR STAFF

The subject of this chapter deserves a great deal of attention from managers and supervisors in the field of aging. Although the chapter contains the last module in the portions of *The Caring Spirit* for professionals, it certainly should not be considered the least important. In fact, it should be at the top of the list when organizing training content for staff.

In the past three decades, researchers have provided professionals in the field of gerontology with a wealth of information about professional and family caregiving. Research has long documented the physical and emotional challenges that professional and family caregivers face. Issues such as caregiver burnout, caregiver burden, and caregiver stress are frequently implicated in the caregiving experiences for both professional and family caregivers.

The professional caregiver research has devoted particular attention to the effects of caregiver burnout and stress on the care of elders. There has been great concern about abuse and neglect of elders because of these factors (Parsons, Simmons, Penn, & Furlough, 2003). Research in this area has focused on the importance of making sure the staff is taught good coping skills and made aware of the red flags that signal burnout, so that abuse, neglect, and burnout can be prevented (Chappell & Reid, 2002).

Although stress and burnout can foster poor care of elders and lead to abuse and neglect, I do not think that this should be the only focus of research. Because there is burnout and stress in this line of work, it is also important to consider how these issues personally affect staff members—emotionally, physically, spiritually, and socially.

The leadership working with staff in long-term care must not lose sight of how this work personally affects staff members and trickles down to all aspects of their lives. Leadership needs to communicate to staff an awareness that the work is stressful and difficult, and that self-care is a priority. Once self-care is acknowledged as a priority, half the battle is won. Thereafter, leadership must provide self-care workshops, places at work for staff members to refresh and replenish themselves, and activities at work that encourage self-care.

DEFINITION OF SELF-CARE FOR CAREGIVERS IN LONG-TERM CARE SETTINGS

Self-care for long-term caregivers requires that staff members take inventory on a regular basis of how they feel physically, emotionally, spiritually, cognitively, and socially. Adhering to self-care discipline places importance on replenishing and nourishing one's spirit and caring for one's soul. It requires awareness, intention, and commitment on the part of the caregiver and the supervisor/manager for the following reasons:

- *Awareness* helps bring forth the issues of self-care that need attention.

- *Intention* helps pave the path for action.

- *Commitment* assures that self-care will be a priority.

In order for staff members to be able to take good care of themselves in the workplace, there has to be a collaborative effort between the staff and leadership. Staff members need to have training that offers the opportunity to learn self-care skills. In addition, the staff should have opportunities to participate in self-care activities at work such as exercise classes, tai chi, yoga, massage, weight management classes, and dance classes.

Following are questions for leadership to consider about recognizing and assessing the need for self-care support in the workplace:

- Does leadership realize the affect caregiving has on the staff's spirits and emotions?

- Does leadership believe self-care is important to the well-being of the staff?

- Is leadership aware of how staff members attempt to take care of themselves in the workplace?

- Has management created ways for staff members to take care of themselves in the workplace?

- Has leadership provided places in the work environment that offer a comfortable, relaxing space for the staff?

- Is leadership willing to allot the time and money it takes to provide training support in this area?

- Is leadership willing to be involved in providing self-care support for staff?

Along with these questions, I have summarized below the most important questions and answers regarding self-care that I have heard from staff members over the years. Their responses are noteworthy and support the need for more attention in this area.

STAFF QUESTIONS AND ANSWERS

1. Do staff members take their breaks and how consistently are they able to do so?

The majority of caregivers say "no," citing reasons such as:

- The facility is often understaffed on their shift, requiring them to care for additional residents. The result is not having enough time to take meals or other breaks.

- The staff working with elders with dementia feel more pressured not to take meal breaks and other breaks because of concern about those residents needing constant supervision from more than one staff member.

- Family members or the elders themselves often interrupt staff members during their meal or other breaks, thus making it difficult to take their breaks.

- Staff members feel they cannot finish all the work they have to accomplish on their shifts, therefore they often do not take their breaks.

2. Do staff members take their vacation time?

There have been mixed responses to this question, including the following:

- Some staff members say absolutely "yes," they know they need to take time off.

- Other staff members say "no," because they need the money and feel they cannot take vacation time.

- A small number of staff members remark about working shifts for their colleagues or helping out friends at their places of work to make extra money during their time off.

3. Are staff members able to find space in their work environments where they can replenish themselves?

The answers to this question tend to have a sarcastic, almost caustic tone, particularly from nursing home caregivers. Answers include the following:

- Most staff members say there is no space in their workplace that is soothing and relaxing.

- Some staff members mention going outside to chill out or take their breaks.

- A few staff members say they sit in their cars, either listening to music or taking a short nap to relax.

4. Do staff members feel leadership supports their efforts to take care of themselves and how?

The majority of staff answer "no" to this question. Responses included the following:

- Most staff members say they do not feel that leadership cares about that.

- Some staff members mention that leadership often rewards them with days off or gift certificates as a way of showing its concern.

5. Do staff members feel that they are given positive, helpful self-care information in their training and are there enough workshops on this topic?

The answers to this question are mixed, and include the following:

- Some staff members feel that workshops on staff burnout and how to cope with stress have been helpful.

- Other staff members feel that the focus was limited to making sure they took care of themselves so that they would take better care of the elders. They do not feel they have learned self-care skills that could personally help them.

- Most mention feeling that they would like to have more workshops on self-care skills.

Comments like this show how important it is to train direct care workers to take care of their own spirits in order to do their work more thoughtfully. Training Module 10 has been designed to do just this.

REFERENCES

Chappell, N.L., & Reid, C.R. (2002). Burden and well-being among caregivers: Examining the distinction. *Gerontologist, 43*(6).

Parsons, S.K., Simmons, W.P., Penn, K., & Furlough, M. (2003). Determinants of satisfaction and turnover among nursing assistants: Results of a statewide survey. *Journal of Gerontological Nursing, 4*(8).

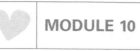 **MODULE 10** # Taking Care of Our Own Spirits

"Before healing others, heal yourself."
—Nigeria, from *A Tiny Treasury of African Proverbs*

INTRODUCTION (10 minutes)

Tools Needed
- Flip chart
- Markers

 Have participants introduce themselves.

 Share with participants the Nigerian proverb above and then ask them what they think it means in relation to the title of this workshop. The trainer should write their responses on the flip chart.

 Share with participants what they should expect to learn from this module and list these on the flip chart.
- Participants will be able to define what self-care in the workplace means.
- Participants will be able to identify ways they sabotage their self-care opportunities.
- Participants will be able to identify barriers to self-care in the workplace.
- Participants will learn at least three *Caring Spirit* ways they can take care of themselves.

 Ask participants if there are any additional expectations they would like to include and write these expectations on the flip chart.

WARM-UP EXERCISE (35 minutes)
"If I Am Not for Myself, Who Will Be for Me?"

Tools Needed
- Flip chart
- Markers
- Handout 10.1

Ask participants to share with the group their definition of self-care in the workplace. The trainer should write their responses on the flip chart.

Ask participants why it is important to take care of themselves. Write their responses on the flip chart. You might want to be sure the following are included:
- If we don't take care of ourselves, then how will we be able to take care of those who need our care?
- Taking care of ourselves helps ensure that we will be better caregivers to those we are caring for and about.
- Taking care of ourselves can help us in the journey of helping those we are caring for to *finish well.*
- Taking care of ourselves helps us have a more realistic, positive perspective.
- Taking care of ourselves is the only way we will be able to care from our hearts.

Ask participants to reflect on what might be some barriers that prevent them from taking better care of themselves in the workplace. Write these responses on the flip chart. You might want to add the following barriers:
- Cultural expectations can prevent us from taking better care of ourselves. If the cultural norm is that women, for example, are expected to be the caregivers of elders, then pressure is placed on the woman to be the primary caregiver. In western culture, the majority of professional and family caregivers are women! Thus, this internalized role can cause guilt in women who do not want to take on this role as the primary caregiver.
- Family expectations can prevent us from taking better care of ourselves. If our family backgrounds have set an expectation that the oldest child in the family is to be the primary caregiver, then that expectation often becomes the norm for that family system.
- In the family therapy field there is a term called *overfunctioner.* An overfunctioner is an individual who believes he or she must be the responsible person for whatever is needed in the family. Overfunctioners are known to have difficulty with setting limits and boundaries and find it difficult to say "no." In the context of professional caregiving, one will

find many caregivers who are overfunctioners in their personal as well as professional lives.

- Our own feelings get in the way; or, as the Buddhists say, our "own self" gets in the way. We become attached to a certain way things ought to be. It then becomes difficult to let go of that perspective. When our feelings get in the way, they can easily cause us to feel guilty, overly responsible, angry, frustrated, or irritated, and we tend not to take good care of ourselves, but instead punish ourselves.
- The workplace does not provide the physical space we need to take better care of ourselves—for example, a place to "chill out," replenish, and just relax.
- Supervisors do not recognize that we are overfunctioning or stressed out, and we may not have found an effective way to tell them what our needs are.

Note: Distribute Handout 10.1 and encourage participants to review the in-depth discussion of self-care included in it.

CORE EXERCISE (25 minutes)
Taking Care of Our Spirits **The Caring Spirit** Way

Share with participants the concept of being *self-full.* Being self-full is a concept for teaching caregivers the importance of intentional, ethical self-care.

Self-full is defined as a way of relating that requires one to consider another person or situation respectfully and thoughtfully but not at the expense of oneself. Being self-full requires one to be aware of personal limits and boundaries. In my work with professional and family caregivers, I rarely come across people who are self-full. Usually they are either selfless or selfish. In this context, a selfless person is one who places everyone's needs before his or her own, and often at his or her personal expense. In fact, when one is selfless, the person's own needs often do not get met at all. A selfish person is one who does not consider others' needs, and at times hurts people's feelings in order to make sure his or her needs are met.

The following is an example of being self-full:

Your co-worker continually asks you to fill in for her. You do so several times, but you notice that it causes you to have to hurry the residents you are responsible for. When your colleague asks you to fill in for her again, you state firmly but kindly that you have helped her several times and that it has made you hurry your own residents. Although you understand her difficulty, you let her know that you cannot help her this time. Remind her that you have helped her out in the past but that you cannot keep on doing so as it places you in an uncomfortable position with your own residents. Thus, in this example, you recognize her dilemma, but you have to take care of yourself, and that is being self-full!

ask

Ask the participants to define ways they can become more self-full in the workplace. Write these on the flip chart. You might want to add the following ways they can be self-full:
- Acknowledging that we have our own limits and boundaries
- Recognizing that we have to advocate for ourselves in sometimes emotionally conflicting circumstances
- Recognizing the needs of the other person and addressing those needs in a nonjudgmental way and with concern, but still holding our position of taking care of ourselves

ask

Have participants divide into small groups. Ask one person from the group to be the recorder. Each participant should share one example of how to implement *The Caring Spirit* way of self-care in the workplace. Each group will then share its comments with the whole group. The trainer should write the responses on the flip chart. The trainer might add the following responses:
- Staff members need to recognize when they need support and ask management for it.
- Staff members need to make sure they take their breaks.
- Staff members need to make room for quiet time at work.
- Staff members could consider bringing spiritual, soothing music to work that they can listen to during their breaks.
- Staff members could give one another shoulder and neck massages.
- Staff members could go outside and focus on the beauty of nature.
- Staff members need to reinforce self-care off the job as well. They need to remember to do the following.
  - Take their vacations
  - Make sure they have *fun* activities in their lives on a consistent basis
  - Participate in religious functions if that helps them take better care of themselves
  - Exercise
  - Eat well, with an emphasis on foods that nourish the soul and body

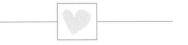

Closing (10 minutes)

Ask the participants to share one new *Caring Spirit* way that they will take better care of themselves. Remind participants to fill out the evaluation forms.

Evaluation Questions

1. Did you find this training helpful? (circle one)   Yes   No
   Please explain why or why not.

   _____
   _____
   _____
   _____

2. Will you be able to use the information
   you learned today at work? (circle one)   Yes   No
   If yes, give at least two examples.

   _____
   _____
   _____
   _____

3. List at least three ways you will take better
   care of yourself after attending this workshop.

   _____
   _____
   _____
   _____

4. Define self care in the workplace.

   _____
   _____
   _____
   _____

5. How did you feel after this workshop? (circle all that apply)

good	encouraged	cared about
sad	bored	listened to
frustrated	informed	angry
blessed	joyful	inspired
motivated	good about myself	

Taking Care of Our Own Spirits
The Caring Spirit™ Way

*"Those who have no compassion for themselves
have none for others either."*
—Rabbi Meir

Staff Questions To Consider

- Do staff members take their breaks and how consistently are they able to do so?
- Does staff members take their vacation time?
- Are staff members able to find space in the workplace to chill-out and replenish?
- Do staff members feel that management supports their efforts to take care of themselves and how?
- Do staff members feel that their training provides positive, helpful self-care information and that there are enough workshops on this topic?

"Before healing others, heal yourself"
—Nigeria, from *A Tiny Treasury of African Proverbs*

Reasons for Self-Care in the Workplace

- If you do not take care of yourselves, then how will you be able to take care of those who need your care?
- Taking care of yourselves helps to ensure that you will be better caregivers to those you are caring for and about.
- Taking care of yourselves can help in the journey of helping those in your care to *finish well.*
- Taking care of yourselves helps you have a more realistic, positive perspective.
- Taking care of yourselves is the only way you will be able to care from your hearts.

Barriers to Self-Care

- Cultural expectations can prevent us from taking better care of ourselves. If the cultural norm is that women, for example, are expected to be the caregivers of elders, then pressure is placed on the woman to be the primary caregiver. In western culture, the majority of professional and family caregivers are women! Thus, this internalized role can cause guilt in women who do not want to take on this role as the primary caregiver.
- Family expectations can prevent us from taking better care of ourselves. If our family backgrounds have set an expectation that the oldest child in the family is to be the primary caregiver, then that expectation often becomes the norm for that family system.

- In the family therapy field there is a term called *overfunctioner.* An overfunctioner is an individual who believes he or she must be the responsible person for whatever is needed in the family. Overfunctioners are known to have difficulty with setting limits and boundaries and find it difficult to say "no." In the context of professional caregiving, we find many caregivers who are overfunctioners in their personal as well as professional lives.
- Our own feelings get in the way; or, as the Buddhists say, our "own self" gets in the way. We become attached to a certain way things ought to be. It then becomes difficult to let go of that perspective. When our feelings get in the way, they can easily cause us to feel guilty, overly responsible, angry, frustrated, or irritated, and we tend not to take good care of ourselves, but instead punish ourselves.
- The workplace does not provide the physical space we need to take better care of ourselves—for example, a place to "chill out," replenish, and just relax.
- Supervisors do not recognize that we are overfunctioning or stressed out, and we may not have found an effective way to tell them what our needs are.

Being Self-full

- Being self-full is intentional, ethical self-care.
- Being self-full is a way of relating that requires us to consider the other person or the situation respectfully and thoughtfully, but not at the expense of ourselves.
- Being self-full requires being aware of our personal limits and boundaries.
- Being self-full acknowledges that we have our own limits and boundaries.
- Being self-full recognizes that we have to advocate for ourselves in sometimes emotionally conflicting circumstances.

Being Selfless

- A selfless person places everyone's needs before his or her own, and often at his or her personal expense.
- A selfless person sometimes does not get needs met at all.

Being Selfish

- Selfish individuals are defined as those who do not consider others' needs.
- At times, selfish individuals will hurt other people's feelings in order to make sure their own needs are met.

Self-Care in the Workplace

- Recognize when you need support and ask management for it.
- Make sure you take your breaks.
- Make room for quiet time at work.

- Bring spiritual, soothing music to work to listen to during your breaks.
- Give one another shoulder and neck massages.
- Go outside and focus on the beauty of nature.
- Reinforce self-care off the job as well. Remember to do the following:
  - Take your vacations
  - Have *fun* activities in your life on a consistent basis
  - Participate in religious functions if that helps you take better care of yourself
  - Exercise
  - Eat well, with an emphasis on foods that nourish the soul and body
  - Spend time with those you love
  - Remember to find reasons to laugh

II

Training for Family Caregivers

11 Why a Spiritual Approach to Caring Matters

"One sees clearly only with the heart.
Anything essential is invisible to the eyes."
—Antoine De Saint-Exupery, from *The Little Prince*

"As we cultivate peace and happiness in ourselves,
we also nourish peace and happiness in those we love."
—Thich Nhat Hanh

"We create our own realities."
—Unknown

OBJECTIVES

- To define *spirituality* in its broadest sense

- To help families understand why integrating a spiritual approach to care can help them feel more comfortable with the care they give their loved ones

- To introduce the Buddhist concept of *beginner's mind* as a way to connect spiritually

A DEFINITION OF SPIRITUALITY

The Caring Spirit approach is unique because the philosophy is based on integrating spiritual concepts and approaches with the provision of care. By embracing this philosophy, families are able to learn how spirituality can help them cope with the challenges they face when caring for their elderly loved ones. In addition, it can help them gain understanding about what spirituality means to their loved ones. Caring from a spiritual perspective can foster connection and help families experience caregiving in a more peaceful and comforting way.

The Caring Spirit definition of spirituality helps families expand their understanding of spirituality. It is defined as a way of being in the world in a trusting, peaceful, faithful, and compassionate state, willing to be open to others with no judgment and being aware of how one connects in the world. For some individuals, spirituality is a path for connecting to God or a higher spirit, thus adhering to a more religious focus. For others, it is a way of connecting to themselves, either through nature or in other sacred and special ways, and thereby revealing the holy. For still others, it is both a religious and personal connection.

Spirituality helps people get in touch with the essence of who they are and how they would like to be in the world. It creates a pathway for people to find meaning and purpose, to make sense of life, and to frame the past, present, and future. When one feels spiritual, one can feel uplifted and honored, respected and valued, cared about and loved.

Helping families to recognize their spiritual sides can result in a more meaningful caregiving experience. Families have shared many stories with me about how they have tapped into their spiritual sides. One daughter simply allowed herself to slow down instead of always feeling that she had to be "doing" for her family member. She said, "When I gave myself permission to just *be* with mom and let go of my constant need to *be doing,* I felt more connected to her and enjoyed my time with her. It was nice to just sit and hold hands."

A son shared remembering as a young child how his mother loved reading Bible stories to him. With some encouragement, he decided to do the same for her. He stated, "When I would read some of the Bible stories Mom read to me, I could see her relax and actually seem to enjoy hearing them read to her. It did not matter if she did not know who I was. What was important was that we were sharing something special together that held meaning for both of us."

A granddaughter shared a touching story about her grandfather, who she loved dearly. He was a farmer and lived most of his life on the farm. When his wife died, he became very depressed. His only daughter lived abroad, but his granddaughter lived in the United States. She encouraged him to move into an assisted living facility near her. With some reluctance, he came. The granddaughter was having a difficult time trying to get him to participate in activities at the assisted living facility. He spent most of his time in his room watching television. After learning about *The Caring Spirit* approach, it occurred to her that she perhaps could bring a little of the farm to him. She contacted a 4H club, which sent a group of young people to assist her grandfather in the construction of a raised garden for the residents. Her grandfather was in charge of making sure all of the plants were watered and harvested at the correct times. She said, "I realized that what Grandpa was missing in his life, besides the best friend he had, his wife, was his love for nature and the earth. This was the way he connected spiritually, and it gave him so much pleasure, joy, and comfort. It also helped him reconnect to others and to me."

One afternoon, I went to visit with my own mother, who has Alzheimer's disease and is living in a nursing home. I could not find her anywhere in the building. I never thought to look in the chapel, until a staff member mentioned that she thought she had seen my mom sitting in there. Well, much to my surprise, my mother was sitting in the chapel. I was surprised because Mom was never a religious person, even though she grew up with some Jewish education. I asked her why she was sitting in the chapel and she clearly and succinctly stated, "I was sitting in here praying to God to ask him why he gave me this Alzheimer's disease. I don't feel like I deserve this and am praying to him to help me."

I was shocked by her answer, but something in me said to try praying together. I held her hand, and we prayed. First we prayed the *Shema,* a sacred Jewish prayer of which she remembered every word. We also prayed that God would help her with her memory. My mother was leaning on her spirituality for comfort, even with her dementia.

There is an important lesson here for families to learn: Do not make the assumption that if a person was not particularly spiritual in earlier life, that he or she will not feel spiritual in later life. Every family member will experience spirituality differently for a variety of reasons. Family backgrounds, individual belief systems, cultural expectations, and one's willingness to be exposed to various spiritual paths all affect one's experience of spirituality.

By learning and following *The Caring Spirit* philosophy, families will increase their awareness of the different ways their members experience spirituality and how spirituality can affect their relationship with their loved one.

MODULE 11 — Why a Spiritual Approach to Caring Matters

"When the eyes see what they have never seen before,
the heart feels what it has never felt."
—Balthasar Gracian

"In the beginner's mind there are many possibilities, but in
the expert's there are few."
—Shunryu Suzuki Roshi, from *Zen Mind, Beginner's Mind*

ask

One week prior to the training session, remind the participants to bring music that makes them feel spiritual.

INTRODUCTION (10 minutes)

> **Tools Needed**
> - Flip chart
> - Markers
> - Handout 11.1

ask

Have participants introduce themselves by asking them the following questions:
- Who are they caring for?
- Is their loved one at home or in a facility?
- How long have they been caring for their loved one?

explain

Share with participants what they should expect to learn from this module and list these expectations on the flip chart.
- Participants will have an understanding of what spirituality means to them.
- Participants will be more aware of what makes them feel spiritual.
- Participants will be more aware of how their family member may experience spirituality.

Note: Distribute Handout 11.1 to participants and encourage them to review the in-depth discussion of finding ways to be more spiritual.

ask

Ask participants if they have other expectations they would like to include, and write their expectations on the flip chart.

WARM-UP EXERCISE (50 minutes)
Listening to Spiritual Music

Tools Needed
- CD or tape player with good speakers
- Flip chart
- Markers

Explain to participants that spirituality can mean different things to different people.
- Spirituality is a way to express one's innermost feelings and emotions.
- Spirituality can open doors to one's self and to one's heart.
- Spirituality is a way to connect with one's past.
- Spirituality is a way to connect deeply to others.
- Spirituality can provide one with a better understanding of another and help him or her to view another with a new *set of eyes.*
- Spirituality helps one to learn how to *be* instead of *doing.*

Ask participants to listen carefully to each piece of music that is presented (play each piece for a minute or two so that participants can get a sense of the piece).

Ask participants to think about
- How the music made them feel
- How the music helped them to connect to the spiritual sides of themselves
- How they might share this music with their loved ones

Ask participants to define spirituality. Encourage them to think about words and values that stem from their own sense of being spiritual. The following list is a sample of words they might choose:

Compassion	Honored	Sacred	Healing
Integrity	Respect	Blessing	Holy
Soul	Joy	Peace	Loving kindness
Heart	Prayer	Uplifted	God, the Lord
Truth	Balance	Honesty	Higher power
Patience	Trust	Spirit	Innermost feelings
Love	Faith	Openness	

Share the following definition of spirituality with the participants: "Being spiritual is a way to get in touch with yourself and to connect to others from the heart and soul. It is a way of *being*, not *doing*, in a more aware and open state. For some, spirituality becomes a path for connecting to God or a higher spirit. For others, it is a way of connecting to the world in a sacred and special way, revealing the holy. It can help you find meaning or purpose, make sense of life, and frame your past. When you feel spiritual, you can feel uplifted, honored, respected, cared for, valued, and loved."

Ask participants how they can be more *spiritual* in the way they care for their loved ones. Following are possible ideas:
- Just *be* with the person, by holding his or her hand or being quiet together
- Read stories or poetry with the person
- Sing to the person
- Cook foods that remind the person of the past or of favorite foods
- Watch joyful movies
- Listen to gospels or other inspirational spiritual music
- Take the person on nature walks or try to bring nature to him or her
- Pray with the person
- Read familiar passages from the Bible, Torah, Koran, or appropriate religious text

Core Exercise (40 minutes)
Developing a Beginner's Mind

> **Tools Needed**
> - Index cards
> - Markers
> - Pens and paper

Share with participants the definition of a beginner's mind:

A beginner's mind is a concept that the Buddhist religion has coined. It is similar to the wonder a child sees in his or her world without preconceptions. A beginner's mind encourages a state of willingness and openness.
- Willingness is defined as being able to let go of the things we cannot control and see things in a different way without judgment.
- Openness is defined as being able to show compassion and to listen in an authentic way.

Share the following with participants: "If we can maintain a beginner's mind, we will be able to stay in the moment, listen from our hearts, and fear less. Our beginner's mind can help us see life's challenges as *growth experiences* instead of *obstacles* to be endured or overcome."

Ask participants to write down on an index card a situation they are experiencing with their loved one or another family member that feels frustrating or difficult. Once they have finished, the trainer should collect the index cards.

Explain to participants that they will take turns reading some of the cards. Utilizing a beginner's mind, ask them to share ways they could cope with the situation or concern. Remind them that by employing a beginner's mind, they are:
- Staying open and willing
- Listening from the heart
- Letting go of what they cannot control
- Being less judgmental
- Showing compassion
- Letting go of the past
- Looking for the possibilities

Explain to participants that it is never easy to deal with situations that feel overwhelming and, sometimes, impossible. If one tries to approach situations with a beginner's mind, however, it encourages options and seeing difficult situations and challenging concerns as *opportunities.*

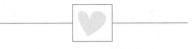

Closing

"Everything in life that we really accept undergoes a change."
—Katherine Mansfield

Share with participants how this quote is about recognizing that life is not static. When we refuse to change and become stuck, we have difficulty with finding options and seeing situations as opportunities. As a result, we can feel sad, depressed, and victimized. The beginner's mind helps us stay open, flexible, and less judgmental. It encourages us to act from our hearts.

Ask participants to fill out the evaluation form.

Evaluation Questions

1. Did you find this training helpful? (circle one)　　　　　　Yes　　　No
   Please explain why or why not.

   _____
   _____
   _____
   _____

4. How would you define a "beginner's mind?"

   _____
   _____
   _____
   _____

2. Do you believe the information in this module will help
   you better tap into your spiritual side? (circle one)　　Yes　　　No
   Please explain why or why not.

   _____
   _____
   _____
   _____

5. How did you feel after this workshop? (circle all that apply)

good	encouraged	cared about
sad	bored	listened to
frustrated	informed	angry
blessed	joyful	inspired
motivated	good about myself	

Spiritual Ways of Caring

*"As we cultivate peace and happiness
in ourselves, we also nourish peace
and happiness in those we love"*
—Thich Nhat Hanh

*"In the beginner's mind there are many
possibilities, but in the expert's there are few"*
—Shunryu Suzuki Roshi, from *Zen Mind, Beginner's Mind*

Spiritual Considerations
- Spirituality is a way to express one's innermost feelings and emotions
- Spirituality can open doors to one's self and to one's heart
- Spirituality is a way to connect with one's past, present, and future
- Spirituality is a way to connect deeply to others
- Spirituality can provide one with a better understanding of another and help him or her to view another with a new set of eyes
- Spirituality helps one to learn how to *be* instead of simply *doing*

Ways caregivers Can Be More Spiritual with Their Loved Ones
- Just *be* with your loved one, by holding his or her hand or being quiet together
- Read stories or poetry with your loved one
- Sing to or with your loved one
- Cook foods that remind your loved one of past favorite foods
- Watch joyful movies together
- Listen to gospels or other inspirational spiritual music
- Take your loved one on a nature walk or try to bring nature to him or her (e.g., bring a bird feeder, bird house, or flowers)
- Pray with your loved one
- Read familiar religious stories or prayers
- Listen to music that your loved one enjoys
- Rub scented cream or hand lotion on your loved ones hands, feet, or shoulders

"Beginner's Mind" Reminders
- Stay open and willing to listen
- Listen from your heart
- Let go of what you cannot control
- Show compassion
- Let go of the way things used to be
- Look for possibilities and opportunities

- Relax your expectations
- Embrace the moment
- Laugh and try to find the humor in things

Helping Families
Connect from the Heart

"I suspect that the most basic and powerful way to
connect to another person is to listen. Just listen. Perhaps
the most important thing we ever give each other is our
attention. And especially if it's given from the heart."
—Rachel Naomi Remen, from *Kitchen Table Wisdom*

OBJECTIVES

- To teach families more effective ways of communicating compassionately with one another and with their loved one(s)

- To help families understand how to encourage a spiritual approach to communication

- To provide spiritual tools families can use for healthier communication

UNIQUE CAREGIVER COMMUNICATION ISSUES

In *Journey of the Heart,* author John Welwood, Ph.D., wrote that it takes a lot of courage to stay honest and open to our own hearts so that we can be honest and open with those we love and care about. He states, "The essence of courage is being willing to feel our heart even in situations that are difficult or painful." Communication can be both painful and difficult, and connecting to our hearts is not easy. It takes a certain amount of courage. Yet, when we are able to communicate from our hearts, it can be meaningful and rewarding. *The Caring Spirit* approach to communication focuses on helping others to connect more to their hearts and find spiritual pathways toward healthier communication.

Communication has mystified and challenged human beings for centuries. Most adults would concur that communication is one of the most difficult facets of their lives. Hundreds of books and seminars are available on the topic of communication. Professionals who counsel clients spend endless hours helping them to become more effective communicators.

Family caregivers have a unique struggle with communication because they interface with many different people. They have to communicate not only with the person they are caring for, but also with other family members, doctors, and various professionals who provide care for their loved one. In addition, they have challenges associated with caregiving that are

- Emotional
- Stressful
- Physically exhausting
- Complex

In my work with family caregivers, I have often heard people talking about these difficulties. Here are just some of their stories:

- A daughter shared, "I find it so difficult to communicate with my siblings. They just don't seem to get it. They complain all the time about mother's care, but when I try to explain to them what is really happening they don't listen and just complain some more. I feel totally frustrated."

- A daughter expressed, "I try to tell my father in the best way I know how that he has to accept some help and he just refuses. He says he doesn't need any help. How do I convince him that he does? I am worried about him being by himself and not getting the care he needs. Plus I am exhausted trying to provide the care he needs."

- A son complained, "I am an only son and child and have my own family that I am responsible for. My kids are small and my wife works as well. I don't know what to do with Dad and Mom. They clearly should not be living alone and yet they refuse to move. I have tried to talk with them and they tell me to mind my own business. Yet, when there is a problem, they expect me to drop everything and come right over."

- A granddaughter shared her frustration, "My grandmother has Alzheimer's disease. My mother refuses to accept that Granny has Alzheimer's disease. When I try to talk with her, she tells me that it is none of my business, it's her mother. I worry about Granny, living all by herself with no help. I don't know how best to talk with Mom. I feel so frustrated and almost angry at Mom."

UNDERSTANDING COMPASSIONATE COMMUNICATION

In her book *Kitchen Table Wisdom,* author Rachel Naomi Remen writes the following about communication:

> I suspect that the most basic and powerful way to connect to another person is to listen. Just listen. Perhaps the most important thing we ever give each other is our attention. And especially if it's given from the heart. When people are talking, there's no need to do anything but receive them. Just take them in. Listen to what they're saying. Care about it. Most times caring about it is even more important than understanding it...
>
> ...Listening is the oldest and perhaps the most powerful tool of healing. It is often through the quality of our listening and not the wisdom of our words that we are able to effect the most profound changes on the people around us. When we listen, we offer with our attention an opportunity for wholeness.

When we communicate from the heart and put our minds aside, we hear and see with commitment and caring. Our communication takes on special meaning. When we listen from our hearts, we pay attention on a deeper level. We listen for understanding, not only for words. We hear the heart and see the soul. This is *authentic* communication.

Authentic communication requires teaching family caregivers to focus on *how* they listen. Professionals might ask them questions such as:

- What does it mean to listen compassionately?

- Do you put your mind aside and listen openly with your heart, without judgment?

- Do you care about what is being said to you?

- Are you comfortable with silence?

- Are you offering your whole attention?

- Do you see listening as an opportunity for understanding and connecting to one another?

Listening is one of the most important skills for effective communication. It is not what one says, but how one is listening that affects communication between people. This is particularly true when caring for elders. Elders have expressed to me that they wish their adult children would "just listen" to them. They are not looking for answers or complete understanding but for compassion and caring. They want to be heard.

This basic need to be heard reinforces the importance of teaching caregivers to use authentic communication.

Listening authentically involves a different set of skills than what people are used to using when communicating. It means helping family members connect first to their own hearts. Family caregivers often have a difficult time staying true to their own hearts because often they are trying to meet everyone else's needs and placing their needs last. Professionals need to encourage family caregivers to pay attention to how they may or may not be listening to their own hearts. It is important to ask the difficult questions, such as:

- Are you being honest with yourself about how you feel?

- Are you taking the time to be quiet and listen to your heart?

- Are you so stressed or exhausted that you can't listen to yourself?

- Are you allowing yourself to be open?

- Are you staying in the moment or being overshadowed by worry or guilt?

Once family caregivers are able to listen to themselves more authentically, professionals need to teach another important spiritual tool: using silence as a way of communicating with those for whom they provide care. Meditation is one spiritual tool that can help to quiet the mind so we can listen more authentically. Professionals can teach meditation techniques as a way to help families learn to be quiet and listen. At the end of Chapter 14 (Handout 14.3) is the Loving-Kindness Meditation adapted from the work of Jack Kornfield, which can be introduced to family caregivers at this stage or when Module 14 is presented.

Western culture values the spoken word. We judge people based on how they communicate verbally. Yet silence can heal and is a powerful way to communicate. Dr. Rachel Naomi Remen shares an important point about silence in her book *Kitchen Table Wisdom:* "Listening creates a holy silence. When you listen generously to people, they can hear truth in themselves, often for the first time... A loving silence often has far more power to heal and to connect than the most well intentioned words."

I attended a workshop on Spirituality and Aging, where Ram Dass was the keynote speaker. I have always considered this man a mentor of mine, someone rich with spiritual wisdom. I had just read his latest book, *Still Here,* written after he had had a stroke that changed his life completely. Being that he was a spiritual person, I was curious about how the stroke might have brought out his spiritual side. I sat on the edge of my chair, anxiously waiting for him to start his talk. He sat in his wheelchair while more than 200 people also anxiously waited to hear what he had to say. He said nothing. He looked around the room and smiled. He must have engaged in this behavior for at least 10 minutes before he finally began to speak. Clearly his stroke had affected his ability to speak. He struggled with a few words, and then he was silent. Sometimes the silence lasted several minutes. The entire talk progressed in the same way. Many people in the audience were squirming in their chairs. They were not used to witnessing this powerful and verbal man struggling with his words and being comfortable with his silence. To me, however, his silence was more powerful than his words ever could be. I hung onto each of his silent moments, letting his words and his silence enter into my heart. I left this powerful workshop feeling very connected to him. I felt his courage, his humility, his spirit, and his connection to my soul.

After this experience, I decided to try a different way of communicating with my own mother. Mom and I had always communicated with one another by talking and discussing whatever was on our minds. With her dementia, communicating with her verbally became difficult. I knew that I needed to find a way to communicate that would still allow us to connect to one another. I decided to see how Mom and I would relate by incorporating silence. Much to my surprise, it was a wonderful way to be with her. We would often sit outside in the garden or inside the nursing home and simply hold hands. We did not need words, because our silence expressed it all. We smiled at one another. I commented on how peaceful it was to be with her this way. She sometimes nodded her head. I truly felt she understood what I was trying to communicate to her without words: that I loved her and I cared about her.

It is important to help families think outside of the box when communicating with their loved one. Even family members who did not have a good relationship with their loved one can try *being together in silence*. They may be amazed how communicating with silence can take some of the pressure off of trying to find something to say, especially when they do not feel like talking or sharing. Other nontraditional ways of communicating may involve using other spiritual tools, such as music, prayer, and touch.

Music is a powerful way to connect people to one another and to their own hearts. Music can open doors that are often closed. For example, I have witnessed elders who were depressed, anxious, or angry show a more peaceful, joyful side of themselves when listening to music. Even elders with dementia can access music. Music touches their hearts in ways that words cannot reach. Listening to music or singing with a loved one can foster a connection that is enjoyable and authentic.

Prayer is another powerful way to communicate with a loved one, particularly if the loved one is comfortable with prayer. When elders are depressed or lonely, it can help to ask them if they are open to praying together. A surprising percentage of elders will agree to do this. Praying together can create a connection that gives the elder a sense of peace, comfort, and hope. Family caregivers who are comfortable with prayer should try this activity with their loved ones.

Last, touch is a wonderful way to communicate. Many elders do not experience as much human touch in their later years. It is amazing how a simple hug or holding a person's hand can communicate feelings and emotions that words cannot express.

The Caring Spirit approach to communication encourages family caregivers to use spiritual approaches to communication. These can have a profound effect on how they communicate with their loved one.

Training Module 12 was developed to help family caregivers recognize the spiritual paths available to help them communicate effectively with all those who are involved in the caregiving process.

REFERENCES

Kornfield, J. (1993). *A Path with heart: A guide through the perils and promises of spiritual life*. New York: Bantam Books

Remen, R.N. (1996). *Kitchen table wisdom: Stories that heal*. New York: Riverhead Press.

Welwood, J. (1990). *Journey of the heart: The path of conscious love*. New York: HarperCollins.

Helping Families Connect from the Heart

> "Sit beside me in long moments of shared solitude,
> knowing both our absolute aloneness and our
> undeniable belonging. Dance with me in the silence
> and in the sound of small daily words, holding neither
> against me at the end of the day."
> —Oriah Mountain Dreamer, from *The Dance*

INTRODUCTION (15 minutes)

> **Tools Needed**
> - Flip chart
> - Markers

ask Have participants introduce themselves. Ask them to share a situation in which they were trying to communicate during the caregiving process and the communication backfired or was misunderstood.

explain Share with participants what they should expect to learn from this module and list these expectations on a flip chart.
- Participants will have a clearer understanding of how to communicate more compassionately and from the heart.
- Participants will learn skills to help them communicate more effectively.
- Participants will be able to recognize some of the barriers to successful communication.
- Participants will learn about spiritual tools for better communication.

ask Ask participants if there are other expectations they would like to include, and write these on the flip chart.

WARM UP EXERCISE (30 minutes)
Roadblocks to Effective Communication

> Tools Needed
> - Flip chart
> - Markers
> - Handout 12.1

Explain to participants that they will learn about some roadblocks to effective communication.

Ask participants to share some of the roadblocks they have experienced while caring for their loved one. Write these examples on the flip chart, and then share the following list of roadblocks to communication:

- Unwillingness to listen: How open are the receiver and sender to listen and not judge?
- Emotional state: Is either the sender or the receiver feeling stressed, depressed, anxious, angry, happy, excited, playful, or tired?
- Attitude: Is the message or information expressed being perceived in a certain way and not in the way it was intended? What type of relationship does the caregiver have with the person he or she is communicating with? Does the caregiver care about how the information is being received? Is the intention or meaning of the message or information carefully considered or said quickly and without much thought?
- Context: Is the appropriate information being delivered for the situation?
- Sensory deficits: Does either the sender or receiver have sensory deficits that make hearing or understanding the information difficult?
- Cognitive deficits: Does either the sender or receiver have cognitive deficits that make understanding the information difficult?

Explain to participants that some communication skills are essential for success. Understanding the process of communication is as helpful as relating from their hearts. Being aware of how others receive the information we share makes an enormous difference to people. It is important to
- Check whether the receiver is able to receive the communication: Is the receiver willing to listen at the time you want to provide the information?
- Check how the information was received by asking the person to repeat what he or she heard
- Pay attention to the receiver's body posture and facial expressions
- Maintain good eye contact

Being clear about what people want to communicate and how they communicate has a significant effect on how the information is understood. It is

essential that when participants communicate with others they pay attention to
- Their own tone of voice
- Their behavior and body language and how it affects the person
- Whether they are communicating compassionately, honestly, gently, and patiently
- How they *connect* to the person with whom they are communicating
- Whether it matters to them if they are understood by the person they are communicating with

Being *prepared* for listening helps participants become more effective communicators when they
- Acknowledge if they are not able to listen at that time
- Recognize how distractions affect their ability to listen
- Listen with their hearts, moving their minds aside
- Do not judge what the person is saying
- Are willing to be silent long enough to truly listen

 Distribute Handout 12.1 and ask participants to review the questions and ponder their answers.

CORE EXERCISE (45 minutes)
Listening from the Heart

> **Tools Needed**
> - Flip chart
> - Markers
> - Handouts 12.2 and 12.3

 Ask the participants what some ways are to communicate compassionately and from the heart? Write their responses on the flip chart.

Afterwards, distribute Handout 12.2 and share the following examples of how they can communicate in *The Caring Spirit* way:
1. *Being compassionate*
   - Listening for understanding, not only for the words
   - Listening patiently instead of hurrying the person
   - Recognizing listening as holy; seeing it as a way to connect deeply and authentically
- Believing that communication is about showing love or caring

2. *Being "true" to oneself*
   - Being *self-full,* which is a term used in *The Caring Spirit* training to define the state of being between selfish and selfless; to be self-full is to make sure you are aware of and take care of your own needs while being sensitive to the needs of your loved one
   - Being honest about what you can and cannot do for your loved one
   - Being honest with your family members about what level of caregiving you can provide

3. *Being willing to communicate in alternative ways*
   - Utilizing other modalities such as music, touch, and prayer to communicate
   - Learning how to *be* with your loved one in a silent connection

Explain to participants that they will have an opportunity to experience some spiritual ways of communicating. Participants will break up into small groups. Each group will be assigned a scenario from Handout 12.3. They are to choose a spiritual way to communicate in response to the scenario. After they decide on their spiritual tools, they will share their way of communicating with the group.

Ask participants to think about the importance of the following:
- Making sure that the *way* they are communicating is understandable.
- Recognizing the effect a relationship can have on communication.
- Examining the nonverbal ways they can communicate.
- Understanding how *caring about* someone changes the way they communicate.

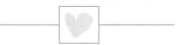

Closing (5 minutes)

Have participants share one way that they will attempt to communicate differently. Express your hope that they have a better understanding of the importance of communicating from the heart.

Ask participants to fill out the evaluation form.

Evaluation Questions

1. Did you find this training helpful? (circle one)　　　　　Yes　　　No
   Please explain why or why not.

   _____

   _____

   _____

2. What are some ways to communicate from the heart?
   Provide at least two examples.

   _____

   _____

   _____

3. What are some of the barriers to communicating with your loved ones?
   List at least two examples.

   _____

   _____

   _____

4. How might you communicate in a more spiritual way?
   List a few examples.

   _____

   _____

   _____

5. How did you feel after this workshop? (circle all that apply)

good	encouraged	cared about
sad	bored	listened to
frustrated	informed	angry
blessed	joyful	inspired
motivated	good about myself	

Helping Families Connect from Their Hearts

"I suspect that the most basic and powerful way to connect to another person is to listen. Just listen. Perhaps the most important thing we ever give each other is our attention. And especially if it's given from the heart."

—Rachel Naomi Remen, from *Kitchen Table Wisdom*

Authentic Communication

What does it mean to listen compassionately?

- Do you put your mind aside and listen openly with your heart, without judgment?
- Do you care about what is being said to you?
- Are you comfortable with silence?
- Are you offering your whole attention?
- Do you see listening as an opportunity for understanding and connecting to one another?

Listening authentically involves a different set of skills. It means connecting to your own heart first. It can sometimes be difficult to stay true to your heart when you are trying to meet everyone else's needs and placing your needs last.

Questions to Ponder

- Are you being honest with yourself about how you feel?
- Are you taking the time to be quiet and listen to your heart?
- Are you so stressed or exhausted that you can't listen?
- Are you allowing yourself to be open?
- Are you staying in the moment or being overshadowed by worry or guilt?

Listening from the Heart...
Toward Spiritual Communication

"Sit beside me in long moments of shared solitude, knowing both our absolute aloneness and our undeniable belonging. Dance with me in the silence and in the sound of small daily words, holding neither against me at the end of the day."
—Oriah Mountain Dreamer, from *The Dance*

Being Compassionate

- Listening for understanding, not only for the words
- Listening patiently instead of hurrying the person
- Recognizing listening as holy; seeing it as a way to connect deeply and authentically
- Believing that communication is about showing love or caring

Being "True" to Oneself

- Being *self-full,* in a state between selfish and selfless; to be self-full is to be aware of your needs and to balance taking care of those needs with being sensitive to the needs of your loved one
- Being honest about what you can and cannot do for your loved one
- Being honest with your family members about what level of caregiving you can provide

Communicating in Alternative Ways

- *Meditation* is one spiritual tool that can help to quiet the mind so you can listen more authentically.
- *Silence* is another way to communicate spiritually—just being in loving silence with your loved one. In her book *Kitchen Table Wisdom,* Rachel Naomi Remen noted the virtues of silence: "Listening creates a holy silence. When you listen generously to people, they can hear truth in themselves, often for the first time... A loving silence often has far more power to heal and to connect than the most well intentioned words." Silence, confirms Remen, can heal and is a powerful way to communicate.
- *Music* is another powerful way to connect people to one another and to connect a person to his or her heart. Music can open doors that are often closed. For example, I have witnessed elders who were depressed, anxious, or angry show a more peaceful, joyful side of themselves when listening to music. Even elders with dementia can access music. Music touches their hearts in ways that words cannot reach. Listening to music or singing with a loved one can foster a connection that is enjoyable and authentic.

- *Prayer* is another powerful way to communicate with a loved one, particularly if the loved one is comfortable with prayer. Prayer can provide a sense of peace, comfort, and hope.
- *Touch* is a wonderful way to communicate. Many elders do not experience as much human touch in their later years. It is amazing how a simple hug or holding a person's hand can communicate feelings and emotions that words cannot express.

Helpful Hints for Successful Communication

- Make sure that the *way* you are communicating is understandable.
- Recognize the effect a relationship can have on communication.
- Examine the nonverbal ways you can communicate.
- Understand how *caring about* someone changes the way you communicate

Listening from the Heart Scenarios

Scenario One

Your mother has Parkinson's disease and is experiencing a lot of physical challenges. She is having difficulty taking a bath, preparing her meals, and dressing because of her tremors. She either needs help in her home or needs to consider moving to an assisted living facility. She has always been an independent woman, however, and has lived in her home for 40 years.

You would prefer that she move into an assisted living facility, however you would be willing to help her find help within her home. When you broach the subject, she refuses to allow a home care companion to come into her home and says she will not ever consider assisted care. She states vehemently, "I can care for myself and I don't want anyone in my home! And I certainly am not moving!"

What might be some ways to *listen from the heart* and communicate more compassionately with her?

Scenario Two

Your father has Alzheimer's disease. Your mother has been trying to take care of him at home but his care is becoming more difficult to manage. He wanders at night, he has urinary incontinence, and he becomes easily agitated. Yet your mother refuses to let you or anyone else help.

What might be some ways to communicate that would convey that you were listening more from the heart?

Scenario Three

Your brother has been caring for your mother in his home. He and his wife are burned out and now want you to take over. Your brother expects you to move your mother into your home, but you know that such a move will not work for your family. When you tell him so, he becomes very angry and accuses you of not caring.

How can you approach him from a *heart full* place?

Spiritual Approaches to Coping with Stress

13

"All it [life] needs is your faithfulness."
—Rachel Naomi Remen, from *My Grandfather's Blessings*

"In our daily lives, we must see that it is
not happiness that makes us grateful,
but gratefulness that makes us happy."
—Albert Clarke

OBJECTIVES

- To reveal how stress affects the way family caregivers cope with caregiving
- To teach spiritual tools to help families cope with the stress of caregiving

RECOGNIZING THE STRESS OF CAREGIVING

Due to advances in medicine, we are able to live longer, fuller, and healthier lives, even individuals with chronic diseases and serious medical conditions. Although this extended lifespan allows families to have more time with one another, it also can mean more complications and stress for families in later life.

With people living longer, many children, spouses, or relatives have had to become the primary caregiver for their elder loved ones. This new role for family caregivers is unfamiliar territory and can cause stress for the caregiver and his or her family. One of the major stresses associated with caregiving is what gerontologists call *role change*. A role change happens when two adults who have interacted with one another on an equal basis experience a change in their relationship because the ill or incapacitated adult is now dependent on the adult who is well. When this role change occurs, there is a shift in roles between the two adults. This role change is stressful and can be fraught with sadness and feelings of being overwhelmed.

It is upsetting, perhaps the greatest sadness that a person can feel, to watch a close family member lose physical and/or cognitive capacity and ability. Adult children often feel that a *role reversal* is occurring as opposed to a role shift. They feel as if they have become the parent and their elder loved one has become the child. Gerontologists disagree with this concept of role reversal, believing it demeans the incapacitated adult and does not take into consideration the difficult emotions that accompany incapacity for the ill elder and the well family member. Helping families acknowledge the stress that is an inevitable part of caregiving is important because it normalizes the experience. Once the family caregiver is able to recognize the different ways stress is affecting him or her, then it becomes important to teach ways to cope with stress. *The Caring Spirit* philosophy to elder care emphasizes a spiritual perspective on stress to help family caregivers approach this challenging time in their lives in a healthier way.

> "Those who have no compassion for themselves,
> have none for others either."
> —Rabbi Meir

THE CARING SPIRIT APPROACH TO STRESS

One might ask, "How can I approach stress from a spiritual perspective when the two words spiritual and stress seem so contradictory?" The word spiritual is often associated with words like calm, peaceful, meditative, inner-focused, or connected. Stress, on the other hand, is associated with words like agitated, anxious, frustrated, or angry. How is it possible that these two words can be complementary when their meanings seem so opposite?

Stress is an inevitable condition that can occur at different times in people's lives, and hundreds of articles and books have been written on the subject, including such topics as

- How to reduce the stress in one's life

- How to remove stress from one's life

- How to cope with stress in the workplace

- Stress-less marriages

- How stress kills

Experts have suggested various ways to eliminate stress. Approaching the issue from a more spiritual perspective presents stress not so much as a problem to be eliminated but as a symptom or reminder that one's soul is not being nourished. When a person's soul is nourished, he or she can think, act, and experience life in a way that moves away from the everyday experiences that tend to annoy, distress, and ultimately stress him or her.

In *Rethinking Alzheimer's Care,* authors Fazio, Seman and Stansell stated, "When people learn to increase their own soulful opportunities and change the way they approach life, they are better able to relate to the people and situations around them." The authors contended that one of the ongoing challenges in life is how to continue to live and act from the soul. To live and act from the soul is particularly difficult when faced with emotional situations that trigger people to feel judgmental or angry, or when they experience differences and grievances that affect them emotionally.

Taking care of a loved one can evoke many emotional responses, and family members often feel as if they are on a continuous seesaw. They do not want to become emotionally anesthetized, yet they find it difficult to cope with the constant emotional upheaval. They feel as if they are living between the sick and the well world.

In addition, some caregivers describe caring for a loved one as living invisibly. In my work with family caregivers, spouses/partners and adult children commented in the following ways about the stress they often feel:

"I sometimes feel so angry and so sad. These emotions often paralyze me. I feel so stressed out that I can hardly think."

"The stress of trying to care for my mother, my children, and my husband is just overwhelming. I feel like I should be able to do it all, but I can't. I am exhausted but know I must keep on going."

"I can never seem to find the time to just enjoy my life. My life is full with making sure dad has his medications, that the staff are following through with what they were hired to do, or running errands for dad. I love him, but sometimes I just resent all the time I have to spend. I want my life back!"

"Because I am the single adult child in the family, my brothers and sisters think I should be the one to take most of the responsibility of caring for Mom. I resent that! I have responsibilities also. Yet, I don't know how to say 'no!' I find that I am so tired and stressed that I have no interest in being with my friends."

When family caregivers become preoccupied with worry, concerns, or guilt, they become stressed and detached from their souls and hearts.

Experts in the field of stress management suggest that the following factors influence the way people manage stress:

- Perception of stress

- Lifestyle

- Personalities

- Family history

- Life situations (work, relationships, finances, or health)

The Caring Spirit approach to stress acknowledges these factors but provides a different perspective on minimizing stress by utilizing a spiritual approach. When people are under stress, they tend to "miss opportunities" as they allow themselves to move out of the moment and become hostage to the situation. They become so stressed out that they deplete their energy.

Training Module 13 was created to help families identify their opportunities to set limits, to view their situations from a different perspective, and to find ways to nourish their souls.

REFERENCES

Fazio, S., Seman, D., & Stansell, J. (1999). *Rethinking Alzheimer's care.* Baltimore: Health Professions Press.

Lerner, H. (1989). *The dance of anger: A women's guide to changing the pattern of intimate relationships.* New York: HarperCollins.

| **MODULE 13** | # Spiritual Approaches to Coping with Stress

"There is often more wisdom to be found at
the edges of life than in its middle."
—Rachel Naomi Remen, from *My Grandfather's Blessings*

INTRODUCTION (15 minutes)

> **Tools Needed**
> - Flip chart
> - Markers
> - Index cards
> - Pens

 Explain to participants that this module will focus on stress and spirituality.

 Share with participants what they should expect to learn from this module and list these expectations on a flip chart.
- Participants will understand how a spiritual approach to stress can be helpful in coping with caregiving.
- Participants will learn spiritual tools for coping with stress.
- Participants will learn ways to nourish their souls.

 Have participants write down on an index card one of the most stressful aspects of caregiving for them. Explain to participants that the cards will be collected and shared later in the training.

WARM-UP EXERCISE (30 minutes)
Help! I'm Sinking in Quicksand!

"There are only four kinds of people in this world...
Those who have been caregivers

Those will be caregivers
Those who are currently caregivers
Those who will need caregivers
—Rosalynn Carter

Tools Needed
- Flip chart
- Markers
- Half the index cards from Introduction
- Handout 13.1

Write the Rosalynn Carter quote on the flip chart. Then, tell participants that there are ways to cope with stress so they do not feel like they are sinking in quicksand. Before caregivers can learn new ways to approach stress from a spiritual perspective, however, they have to be able to set limits. Distribute Handout 13.1 and discuss its contents.

Limit setting is not easy and takes a great deal of practice. In fact, it can be compared with learning to drive a car. Anyone who knows how to drive remembers having to take driving lessons and practice driving. The same learning process holds true for learning to set limits. Caregivers can easily feel overwhelmed when trying to find time to care for their loved one and also care for themselves. They often place their needs last. Even a passage in the Bible reminds us: "If I am not for myself, who will be for me?" Caregivers, however, have a hard time adhering to that passage.

Dr. Harriet Lerner, author of *The Dance of Anger,* said that limit setting has always been difficult, particularly for women. Learning how to set appropriate limits, however, is crucial to coping more effectively with stress. Following are some suggestions on how to set limits while caregiving:

- Be aware of what your needs and limits are. This can be tricky because caregivers often express feeling guilty or selfish if they think of themselves.
- Make sure to communicate to your family what you can and cannot do.
- Remember to ask for professional help when you feel overwhelmed or emotional. Consider going to a professional who can provide unbiased help in determining the needs of both the caregiver and the loved one.
- Be willing to ask others for help. For example, a grandson could run errands or stay with your loved one while you run the errands. You could also occasionally ask a neighbor to make a meal to relieve you of this task.
- Recognize that all family members must be taken into consideration when setting limits, not just the elder and caregiver. Know that you can not always make everyone happy. Instead, keep focused on finding the best possible solution to the problem or concern at hand.

Give participants the opportunity to practice limit setting with some of the situations they wrote down on their index cards. In their responses, ask them to consider some of the suggestions that you have shared. Encourage them to refer to Handout 13.1.

Explain to participants that once they have a good understanding of setting limits, they can begin to focus on how to implement spiritual tools for coping with stress.

CORE EXERCISE (30 minutes)
Taking Care of Our Own Spirits **The Caring Spirit** Way

Tools Needed
- Flip chart
- Markers
- Half the index cards from Introduction
- Handout 13.2

Explain to participants that they will engage in a short group discussion on the differences between having a *soulful experience* versus a *stressful experience* when caring for a loved one. Discuss the table in Handout 13.2.

Share with participants that they will now have an opportunity to apply some of the concepts they just discussed. With the remaining index cards, have participants apply a more spiritual perspective to coping with the stressful scenarios.

Ask participants to share ways they currently cope spiritually. After they share their responses, mention any additional responses from this list:
- Praying
- Attending church or synagogue
- Participating in soothing activities for the soul, such as massage, tai chi, yoga, or meditation
- Activities that connect them to nature, such as gardening, nature photography, walking in parks, hiking, or camping
- Focusing on breathing by simply slowing down and taking deep breaths when stressed
- Singing
- Dancing

Closing (15 minutes)
Ask the Angels

> **Tools Needed**
> - Handout 13.3 (copy and cut out the set of Angel Cards in this handout)
> - A box for the Angel Cards

Reinforce for participants that it is not easy being a caregiver and experiencing their loved one's decline. Drawing on their spiritual sides is a way to "keep the faith."

In today's society, angels are often looked upon as sources of strength and courage, providers of support, and messengers of hope. Whether participants believe in angels as spirits or beings does not matter. What is important is that in today's society, angels are cherished, and they hold positive meaning in American culture. Most people have experienced an angelic moment, perhaps when they witnessed the birth of a child, a shooting star, a beautiful rainbow, or a person's last breath. Some people have even had a near-death experience from which they were rescued by "an angel."

The following optional exercise can help caregivers cope with the difficult task of caregiving. It leaves caregivers with a comforting yet tangible spiritual tool that can be used on a daily basis.

Explain to participants that they will have an opportunity to ask the *angels* what they might need to help them cope with their caregiving experience. Tell them that each participant will pick one angel card.

Note: if the group is too big for everyone to pick a card, call on a few participants from the group to pick cards.

After each participant picks a card, he or she is to share the card they picked with the group and think about *why* he or she got that particular card. For example:
- If a participant picks the card that says "understanding," the trainer might ask why he or she might need that quality in his or her current caregiving experience. Ask the participant to explore the reasons why he or she may need to demonstrate understanding at this time.
- If a participant picks the card "honesty," ask him or her, "Do you see honesty as important to your current caregiving experience?"

Note: This can be an emotional exercise for participants. If a participant reveals emotions that are upsetting to him or her, the trainer needs to help the participant process them. The trainer, when appropriate, should encourage the participants to share similar experiences so that the person may not feel so alone. If it seems that the person is overwhelmed, ask him or her to stay after the session so that you can talk with him or her. It might be

appropriate to suggest a family counselor who works with people struggling with caregiving issues.

ask Have the participants fill out the evaluation form.

Evaluation Questions

1. Did you find this training helpful? (circle one)　　　　　Yes　　　　No
    Please explain why or why not.

    _____

    _____

    _____

2. Do you believe you will cope with stress differently
    after participating in this workshop? (circle one)　　　Yes　　　　No
    Please explain why or why not.

    _____

    _____

    _____

3. What are some *barriers* to communicating with your loved ones?
    List at least two examples.

    _____

    _____

    _____

4. What might be some ways to cope with stress with a more spiritual approach?
    List a few examples.

    _____

    _____

    _____

5. How did you feel after this workshop? (circle all that apply)

good	encouraged	cared about
sad	bored	listened to
frustrated	informed	angry
blessed	joyful	inspired
motivated	good about myself	

Setting Limits to Reduce Stress

When family caregivers move from "being in the moment" to "being preoccupied with worry and concerns or guilt," they become stressed and subsequently detached from their souls and hearts. *The Caring Spirit* philosophy provides a different perspective on how professionals can help families take care of themselves utilizing a spiritual approach.

The following factors influence the way people manage stress:
- Perception of stress
- Personality
- Life situations (i.e., work, relationships, finances, health)
- Lifestyle
- Family History

Learning to set limits is a prerequisite to learning new ways to approach stress from a spiritual perspective. Limit setting is not easy and is much like learning to drive a car: It takes a lot of practice before it comes easily. Caregivers can easily feel overwhelmed when trying to find time to care for their loved one and also for themselves. They often place their own needs last. A passage from the Bible reminds us: "If I am not for myself, who will be for me?"

 Harriet Lerner, author of *The Dance of Anger,* said that limit setting has always been difficult for people, especially for women. Learning how to set appropriate limits, however, is crucial to coping more effectively with stress. Following are some suggestions for how to set limits while caregiving:
- Be aware of your needs and limits. This can be tricky, because caregivers often express feeling guilty or selfish if they think of themselves.
- Make sure to communicate to your family what you can and cannot do.
- Remember to ask for professional help when you feel overwhelmed or too emotional. Consider going to a professional who can provide unbiased help in determining the needs of both the caregiver and the loved one.
- Be willing to ask others for help. For example, a grandson could run some errands or stay with your loved one while you run the errands.
- Recognize that all family members must be taken into consideration when setting limits, not just the elder and the caregiver. Know that you cannot always make everyone happy. Instead, keep focused on finding the best possible solution to the problem or concern.

Soulful Versus Stressful Experiences

Soulful Experience	Stressful Experience
Experience the moment	Worry about what might happen or has not happened
Come more from the heart, using intuition and feeling	Stay in the head, using judgment and ego
Appreciate all the abundance in your life	Focus on what you don't have and think about things in a negative way
Recognize the inner beauty of people and things; see a "crisis" as an *opportunity,* see a "failure" as a *learning experience*	Focus on what you don't like about a person; see a situation as a failure or terrible crisis
Love unconditionally	Love only because you want approval or seek to please someone
Be still and quiet	Stay busy and constantly doing something
Be open and willing to be flexible or to give up control	Believe things are to be done only your way and stay *task-centered* instead of *heart-centered*
Acknowledge and express anger appropriately	Hold in your anger until you explode or get sick
Be kind and gentle to yourself	Be hard on yourself and punish yourself by overeating, drinking alcohol, or participating in other harmful behaviors

Angel Cards
(Copy and cut apart)

forgiveness	education	faith	delight
surrender	healing	courage	trust
flexibility	patience	strength	birth
balance	obedience	love	joy
responsibility	release	clarity	gratitude
purpose	willingness	power	humor
compassion	adventure	purification	freedom
expectancy	creativity	beauty	honesty
enthusiasm	responsibility	understanding	synthesis
efficiency	abundance	peace	light
simplicity	inspiration	openness	truth
tenderness	transformation	play	grace
integrity	communication	harmony	spontaneity
sisterhood/ brotherhood			

Helping a Family Member Finish Well

"Our pleasures are shallow, our sorrows are deep."
—Cheyenne Indian tribe, from *The Soul Would Have No Rainbow if the Eyes Had No Tears*

"Befriending life often requires
accepting and experiencing loss."
—Rachel Naomi Remen, from *My Grandfather's Blessings*

OBJECTIVES

- To define for family members the concept of *finishing well*

- To understand the normal stages of the grieving process along with anticipatory grieving

- To highlight different spiritual ways of coping with loss

UNDERSTANDING LOSS

Advanced age and chronic illness brings many losses. Some families experience these profound losses as life-altering experiences full of great meaning and value. Other families may experience the same loss as devastating, bringing great suffering and overwhelming sadness. As Judith Viorst, author of *Necessary Losses*, suggested, "As long as we are living we will experience lifelong losses." She called these losses the "necessary losses" of life, saying, "These losses are universal, unavoidable, inexorable." She claimed that central to understanding life is our understanding of how we deal with loss. Stephen Levine, author of the book *A*

Year to Live, embraced the same philosophy. He suggested that we "practice our dying." By "practice," he meant that we continually need to reevaluate what our lives mean to us. By practicing our dying, we remember that life is tenuous and not to be taken for granted. He suggested that we consider some of the following questions as a way of practicing our dying:

- Have we dealt with our *unfinished business,* or the business of life that we need to find some closure around?

- Are we continually looking for the possibilities of life, the opportunities that can help us to grow?

- Do we live in the present and allow ourselves to learn from our past? Or do we hold onto life and the past in a way that causes us continued suffering?

- Do we live in our heart or in our head?

- Are we committed to living a life that is more fully alive?

Professionals can ask some of these questions as a way of helping families consider the way loss affects their lives. Asking families to reexamine what each loss represents to them can help them gain a fresh perspective that provides them with the opportunity to learn and grow from their experience.

> "And ever has it been that love knows not
> its own depth until the hour of separation."
> —Kahlil Gibran, from *The Prophet*

The death of a loved one is one of the most profound losses a person will experience. For many caregivers, the grief that accompanies loss is multifaceted and can be complicated. Following are some reflections families have shared about how they feel about the impending loss or the death of their loved ones:

> "I love my mom dearly but am at a point where I am just tired. Tired of visiting her at the nursing home, tired of seeing her lose capacity, tired of being tired. Sometimes I secretly wish she would die. Yet, I love her and would miss her so."

> "My sister and I have very different feelings about our mother. We always have. I want to do everything I possibly can to keep Mom comfortable. Whatever it takes, I will make it happen. My sister, on the other hand, states that her number one priority is her own family. So she often is not available when things get tough. That makes me very angry. I just don't understand her."

> "My father was my role model and mentor. He helped me start my business. Now he is very sick. He has chronic obstructive pulmonary disease (COPD) and is on oxygen 24 hours a day. He can do very little for himself. We have a caregiver with him during the day, but not at night. Money is tight. I stay there every night to make sure he is okay. I try to explain to my wife that this is just a temporary situation, but she refuses to under-

stand and is angry with me. Yet she never had a good relationship with either of her parents. "

"My mom has Alzheimer's disease. I hate seeing what is happening to her. She is incontinent, cannot walk anymore, and is having trouble with her speech. It makes me so sad, I can hardly stand visiting with her at the nursing home. Each time I leave I feel so depressed. It stays with me for days. I just don't know how to live with her disease."

Researchers in the field of bereavement and grief say that the process of letting go is a normal and important part of life, especially at the end of life. Losses are better tolerated when there is an opportunity to say goodbye. Professionals need to encourage family caregivers to share their grief and sadness with others, yet this process of sharing can sometimes be difficult if the family member is in denial or is uncomfortable with expressing feelings. Often the best counsel that a professional can offer is education about the grieving process and resource materials.

UNDERSTANDING ANTICIPATORY GRIEVING AND THE GRIEVING PROCESS

It takes great courage and love to say goodbye to a family member. Families often experience what is called *anticipatory grieving,* which is the process by which family members begin to let go and say goodbye to their loved one while the person is still alive. This process involves acknowledging the impending death and recognizing the unfinished business they still have to sort through to attain some closure. It involves recognizing the role their loved one played in their lives and finding ways to acknowledge how much that role meant. Often family members are recognizing that the person is no longer the person they knew because of severe physical or cognitive decline. Professionals need to help family caregivers understand that anticipatory grieving is a normal part of the grieving process. Many of the same stages of grieving that occur when someone dies can occur during this process as well.

Elisabeth Kübler Ross, authority on death and loss and author of *On Death and Dying,* identified five stages of grieving that she believed individuals experience with an impending death or actual death. Professionals now know that people do not necessarily experience these stages in a certain order as Ross had thought. Some may skip a stage or even experience all of the stages and then go back to one of them later on. The stages of grieving, which can also be experienced in anticipatory grieving, are:

1. **Shock and Denial:** In this stage, family members are given the diagnosis that their loved one has a terminal illness. The diagnosis can bring forth shock, denial, or both, because the information can be overwhelming and hard to digest, especially in the beginning. Usually after a family has had some time to process the information, its members are able to move forward and acknowledge the impending loss.

2. **Bargaining:** In this stage, the family recognizes that death is imminent or will happen over time and feels the need to hold onto the hope that if they pray, or act in a different way, their family member won't die.

3. **Anger:** In this stage, family members are upset and angry that their loved one is going to die. There are a number of ways that anger can be expressed, such as being verbally angry at the person that is ill, venting their anger on others, or internalizing their anger, which can result in the next stage, depression.

4. **Depression:** In this stage, family members may process their sadness and experience a number of emotions that result in depression. They tend to feel hopeless and overwhelmingly sad, and they may find it difficult to concentrate and care for their family member.

5. **Acceptance:** In this stage, family members are able to recognize that loss is inevitable and can give themselves permission to move forward.

It is important for families to understand that it is not unusual to experience anticipatory grieving when they are caring for a loved one. Professionals need to inform families that a wide range of emotions—ranging from guilt, anger, profound sadness and depression to relief—can accompany anticipatory grieving.

Anticipatory grieving affects how families cope with saying goodbye. If they do not accept the impending loss of their loved one, they often do not experience anticipatory grieving. However, if they are able to acknowledge the impending loss of their loved one, professionals can help them cope with this loss.

Some additional factors can affect the process of saying goodbye for family caregivers:

1. The relationship between the family caregiver and loved one; this can determine the level of difficulty or ease in letting go

   • For some there may be unfinished business—emotional concerns that have never been addressed.

   • For others, there may have been inappropriate boundaries between the family member and his or her loved one that have existed for most of the relationship.

2. The loved one's own awareness of his or her condition and readiness to let go

   • If the loved one is in denial, it can be hard for family members to process their grieving.

   • If the loved one has accepted his or her condition, it may ease the family's grieving process.

3. The family members' own feelings about death and loss

   • How family members feel about death and loss can affect their ability to let go of their loved one and eventually accept their loved one's death.

- If family members are afraid of death and loss, or are unwilling to acknowledge it, they can become stuck in the grieving process.

- How willing family members are to let go of their loved one will greatly affect the grieving process.

4. Whether the family and the loved one have religious or spiritual supports

- Researchers have found that when people are positively connected to their religion or spiritual beliefs, they work through the grieving process with less stress and depression.

- Families who do not have any spiritual support may have a difficult time accepting the death and moving forward in the grieving process.

It is important for professionals to realize that saying goodbye can be a complicated process. Helping families through this maze of experiences and emotions is essential to good care.

HELPING FAMILIES FINISH WELL

> "People die, but love does not die.
> It is recycled from one heart, from one life, to another."
> —Rabbi Harold Kushner, from *Living a Life that Matters*

Family therapist Terry Hargrave coined the term "finishing well," which refers to helping elders and their families find a sense of connectedness and peacefulness at the end of their lives. Finishing well also can help families recognize the legacies that their loved one may leave for the family and community.

One of the best ways for professionals to help families come to terms with finishing well is through an approach called *life review*, which can be used to review and examine the meaning of their lives. Families and their loved ones can be involved in the life review process by asking the following questions, which have been divided into questions for the elder and questions for family members.

For the Elder

1. What aspects of your life held the most meaning for you?

2. What legacy might you leave for your families?

3. What legacy might you leave for the community?

4. What were some of the experiences in your life that filled you with joy?

5. What would you like to say to your family and friends before you die?

For Family Members

1. What would you like to know about your loved one that you feel you don't know?

2. What has your loved one meant to you?

3. Is there some unfinished business you need to take care of before your loved one is gone?

Even elders who have Alzheimer's disease or other forms of dementia can use life review to find a sense of connectedness and to finish well. Professionals should suggest the following ideas to family members to help stimulate the life review process:

• Share pictures of family, friends, and pets.

• Bring in familiar memorabilia about their lives (e.g., items from work, hobbies, interests).

• Have them listen to music, which not only brings back memories but often also is calming and soothing.

• Share foods and engage in cooking activities to stimulate memory.

Another way professionals can help family members finish well is to consider engaging the services of hospice. Hospice is a service that helps people who are terminally ill have a pain-free end of life and a dignified death. The goal of hospice professionals is to provide comfort and care to the dying individual and to provide support to family members. The hospice team typically includes a social worker, pastoral professional, nurse, nursing assistant, medical director, and volunteer. Most nursing homes either have a contract with a hospice program or will allow the family to contract with one.

A frequently asked question is how families know when it is time for their family member to be placed in hospice care? The following are some suggestions that professionals can offer families to consider:

• If their family member has a terminal illness or is in the end stages of their disease, he or she is probably an appropriate candidate for hospice care.

• Hospice care treats not only people with cancer, but also patients with all types of end-stage illnesses, such as Alzheimer's disease, Parkinson's disease, chronic obstructive lung disease, and so forth.

• If their family member lives in a long-term care facility encourage family members to consult with the facility's director of nursing or the charge nurse for advice. They are usually good at knowing when someone is nearing the end of his or her life, based on the resident's presenting symptoms.

• Make sure the family communicates to the family member's doctor the concern that hospice care might be needed. Quite frequently, unless their patient has cancer, doctors forget to think about prescribing hospice care.

- Remind family members that they often have to be an advocate for their family member. If their loved one lives in a long-term care facility, the staff and the doctor sometimes do not think about using hospice for residents. Do not hesitate to bring the possibility of hospice care to their attention. Hospice can be a great resource and wonderful support for all concerned, including the staff.

SPIRITUAL WAYS OF COPING WITH LOSS

> "Wisdom requires that we relax our hold on our picture of how things 'ought' to be and learn to make peace with things as they are. We can only do this moment by moment, here and now, by responding with open hearts and minds to the changes that occur."
> —Ram Dass, from *Still Here*

> "To love fully and live well requires us to recognize finally that we do not possess or own anything—our homes, our car, our loved ones, not even our own body. Spiritual joy and wisdom do not come through possession but rather through our capacity to open, to love more fully, and to move and be free in life."
> —Jack Kornfield, from *A Path with Heart*

In the past few years, as I have worked with families and helped them cope with loss, I have found that there is a need to think differently about how we value elders and the end of life. One of the best ways for professionals to help families cope with loss and finish well is to encourage families to frame their thinking about loss differently.

Ram Dass, author of *Still Here* and authority on Eastern thinking, supports the notion that Western culture's belief about *finishing well* has more to do with "the stuff of the ego" than with "spirit and soul." He defined *ego* as the self that is outer-focused, so that "ego includes all the things we experience on the psychophysical plane." According to Dass, ego is about how we dress, our outer selves, how we want people to think about us, what we want people to believe about us, our possessions, and our fame. The ego is the *who* we think we are. In essence, we become actors in our own lives.

Dass claimed our ego experiences aging and death as something to dread, something that grips us and should be ignored. Western culture subscribes to and values the concept of ego. A successful life in Western culture is defined as a life that is productive, that has accumulated wealth and material things. Independence is highly valued and interdependence or dependence is viewed as being a "burden." Ram Dass believes Western culture's way of thinking creates challenges for elders and their families to finish well. He called these challenges "attachment to suffering." He expressed that as long as people value the "stuff of the ego they will suffer." This suffering results in families having a difficult time saying goodbye to their loved ones, seeing their loved ones as burdens, and having difficulty working through the stages of grieving.

Other cultures hold beliefs similar to those of Ram Dass regarding old age and the end of life. Native American and African cultures have rich traditions and beliefs about finishing well. Their focus is on recognizing the accomplishments of their elders and respecting those contributions. The expectation of old age is that elders serve as reminders to the young of how important the lives of their elders have been to their culture.

In her book *Another Country*, author Mary Pipher also expressed the belief that western culture needs to change its focus on how elders are valued. She claimed that so much of what she has learned about herself and her life has been through connecting with the elders in her family. She reminds us of a quote from Alex Haley that serves as a powerful metaphor about elders: "The death of an old person is like the burning of a library." She noted that "visiting my aunts allowed me to read some of the books before they burned."

Building on the power of this metaphor, I would like to propose that the usual coping strategies currently used to help families are not adequate. Professionals can help elders and their families not to cling so strongly to western beliefs and to adopt other ways of thinking about the end of life. To do so, they will need to provide families with a variety of ways to cope.

Training Module 14 teaches families some spiritual approaches to coping and helps them understand this sacred last stage of life so that they too have the opportunity to finish well.

REFERENCES

Dass, R. (2000). *Still here: Embracing aging, changing and dying.* New York: Riverhead books.

Gibran, K. (1923). *The prophet.* New York: Alfred A. Knopf.

Hargrave, T.D., & Anderson, W.T. (1992). *Finishing well: Aging and reparation in the intergenerational family.* New York: Brunner/Mazel.

Kübler-Ross, E. (1997). *On death and dying.* New York: Scribners.

Levine, S. (1997). *A year to live: How to live this year as if it were your last.* Boston: Beacon Press.

Pipher, M. (1999). *Another country: Navigating the emotional terrain of our elders.* New York: Riverhead Books.

Viorst, J. (1986). *Necessary losses: The loves, illusions, dependencies, and impossible expectations that all of us have to give up in order to grow.* New York: Ballantine Books.

| **MODULE 14** | # Helping a Family Member Finish Well

"Old age offers the opportunity to shift our
cares away from the physical toward what cannot
be taken away: our wisdom and the love wc offer
to those around us. But a culture without spiritual
underpinnings deprives us of this opportunity"
—Ram Dass, from *Still Here*

INTRODUCTION (10 minutes)

> **Tools Needed**
> - Flip chart
> - Markers

ask

Have participants introduce themselves.

explain

Share with participants what they should expect to learn for this module and list those expectations on the flip chart.
- Participants will be able to define the concept of *finishing well.*
- Participants will be more aware of their own fears about *letting go* and recognize they are not alone in those fears.
- Participants will be able to define anticipatory grieving and become aware of the feelings and emotions involved in this process.
- Participants will learn some spiritual tools to help them cope with the end of life.

explain

Share with participants the quote at the beginning of the module. Ask them what they think this quote means. The trainer might add that the quote offers the following:
- A different way for participants to experience their loved ones' aging
- A different way for participants to show they care by connecting in spiritual ways
- A different way for elders to view their own aging

195

"The soul would have no rainbow if the eyes had no tears."
—Minquass Indian tribe saying, from *The Soul Would Have No Rainbow if the Eyes Had No Tears*

WARM-UP EXERCISE (30 minutes)
Anticipatory Grieving: The Long Goodbye

> Tools Needed
> * Handout 14.1
> * Index cards containing different feelings (see Note below)
> * Numbers

Note: Prior to the start of this training session, the trainer should write the following words describing possible feelings of caregivers on a set of index cards:

Anger	Despair	Depressed
Sadness	Shame	Denial
Frustration	Embarrassment	Acceptance
Lonely	Exhaustion	
Guilt	Anxious	

Share with participants the concept of anticipatory grieving. Mention that they should refer to Handout 14.1.

Explain to participants that they will play a game that will help them identify feelings that are associated with anticipatory grieving. Each person will be given a number. The person who picks the largest number will go first. This person will pick one index card that will have a word that expresses a feeling. He or she is to consider whether that word is a feeling being experienced as his or her loved one becomes more frail. If the person cannot relate to the feeling, the card can be placed back in the pile and another card selected. As each participant picks a card, he or she is to address that feeling and share it with the group. The last person can pick either the last card or trade his or her card for someone else's card.

After everyone has had the opportunity to share, the trainer might want to ask participants how the game helped them understand the feelings associated with anticipatory grieving.

CORE EXERCISE (45 minutes)
Letting Go Isn't So Easy to Do!!!

*"When you are sorrowful look again in your heart
and you shall see that in truth you are weeping
for that which has been your delight"*
—Kahlil Gibran, from *The Prophet*

Tools Needed
- Flip chart
- Markers
- CD player
- Handouts 14.2 and 14.3
- Soothing music for "Loving-Kindness Meditation"

 explain
Share with participants the quote at the beginning of this exercise. Ask them what is meant by the quote, particularly as it relates to their personal situations. Why do they think it is so hard in our culture to let go of those we love? The trainer should write some of the answers on the flip chart.

Share with participants Handout 14.2. The trainer should have each participant read one barrier from the handout.

 ask
Ask participants to join up with one or two other participants. They are to share with each other their biggest fears about *letting go* of their loved one. Then have the whole group discuss some of the fears shared within the small groups. The trainer should write these fears on the flip chart.

 ask
Ask participants to think of some ways to work through the barriers of letting go. They can refer to the handout with suggestions on working through barriers.

explain
Tell participants they will have an opportunity to practice a spiritual approach to letting go. They will learn a meditation that can help calm their minds, soothe their hearts, and help them practice letting go.

Participants need to get comfortable, either in chairs or on the floor. The trainer will take them through a meditation. If any participants do not wish to join in the exercise, then they may observe.

ask
Afterward ask participants if the meditation helped them become more comfortable in any way with the idea of letting go and saying goodbye. Write on the flip chart what the experience was like for the participants.

Note: Distribute Handout 14.3 describing the Loving-Kindness Meditation and suggest participants practice it on their own whenever they wish.

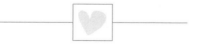

Closing (5 minutes)

 explain
Share with participants that you hope they have learned some new ways to cope with anticipatory grieving and to use these to help them *finish well*. Have participants fill out the evaluation form.

Evaluation Questions

1. Did you find this training helpful? (circle one)   Yes   No
   Please explain why or why not.

   _____
   _____
   _____

2. Will you be able to use the information
   you learned today? (circle one)   Yes   No
   Please give a few examples.

   _____
   _____
   _____

3. Was it helpful to learn about anticipatory grieving and the stages of grieving?
   Please share a few reasons.

   _____
   _____
   _____

5. How did you feel after this workshop? (circle all that apply)

good	encouraged	cared about
sad	bored	listened to
frustrated	informed	angry
blessed	joyful	inspired
motivated	good about myself	

Anticipatory Grieving
and Stages of Grieving

It takes great courage and love to say goodbye to a family member. Anticipatory grieving is the process by which family members begin to let go and say goodbye to their loved one. This process involves:

- Acknowledging the impending death
- Identifying any unfinished business (stuff you have been ignoring or have attempted to push away from your mind)
- Recognizing the role your loved one played in your life and finding ways to acknowledge what that role meant
- Recognizing that your loved one might not be the person you remembered him or her to be; learning to accept that person as he or she is now
- Recognizing the stages of grieving you may go through and allowing yourself to go through them

Stages of Grief

1. Shock and Denial
   - In this stage, you have learned for the first time that your loved one has a terminal illness. The diagnosis can bring forth feelings of shock, denial, or both because the information can be overwhelming and hard to digest.
   - Usually, after you have had some time to process the information, you are able to move forward and acknowledge your impending loss.

2. Bargaining
   - In this stage, you recognize that death is imminent or will happen over time.
   - You may hold onto hope that maybe if you pray hard enough, or act in a different way, your family member will get better or won't die.

3. Anger
   - In this stage, you are upset and angry that your loved one is going to die. There are a number of ways that anger may get expressed:
     - Becoming verbally angry at the person
     - Venting your anger on others
     - Internalizing your feelings, which can result in depression or even physical illness

4. Depression
   - In this stage, you feel sadness and experience a number of emotions that can result in depression.
   - You may feel hopeless or overwhelmingly sad, and may find it difficult to concentrate and take care of your family member or even yourself and others.

5. Acceptance
   - In this stage, you are able to recognize that the loss is inevitable and you give yourself permission to move forward.

Barriers to Letting Go

History of Relationships

The relationship between the family caregiver and his or her loved one can determine the level of difficulty or ease in letting go.

- For some people there may be unfinished business—emotional concerns that have never been addressed.
- For others, there may have been inappropriate boundaries between the family member and his or her loved one that have existed for most of the relationship.

Awareness of Condition

The level of awareness that a loved one has of his or her condition and the readiness to let go that he or she expresses can affect how family members feel.

- If their loved one is in denial, it can be hard for the family members to process grieving.

Feelings About Death and Loss

How family members feel about death and loss can affect their ability to let go of their loved one and eventually accept their loved one's death.

- Individuals who are afraid of death and loss or are unwilling to acknowledge it can become stuck in the grieving process.
- How willing family members are to let go of their loved one greatly affects the grieving process.

Religious Beliefs

The existence or lack of religious or spiritual supports, for either family members or their loved one, can play a large role in how grief and loss are processed.

- Researchers have found that when people are positively connected to their religion or spiritual beliefs, they work through the grieving process with less stress and depression.

Loving-Kindness Meditation

Meditation is a way for individuals to connect to themselves and to their hearts in a quiet, intentional, and loving way. When meditating, you only need a place that is comfortable so you can quiet your mind and connect to the heart. The Loving-Kindness Mediation was developed by Jack Kornfield, author of the book *A Path with Heart,* as a way to help people slow down, let go of the stress in their lives, and realize the abundance and love in life.

When you sit down to try the meditation, make sure you have the time and quiet space simply to *be* with yourself and your surroundings, uninterrupted by children, grandchildren, spouses, neighbors and so forth.

Find a place to relax fully, whether in a favorite chair, in a garden, on a porch, or on a couch. Close your eyes and take deep breaths. Breathe in and then breathe out, listening to your breathing and being quietly attentive to it. Listen also to your heartbeat. It is amazing what our bodies do every day that we pay little attention to and take for granted. Then, in you head or out loud, say the Loving-Kindness Meditation below.

If you try this meditation daily, it might give you an opportunity to get more in touch with what is truly important in your life. It surely will slow you down even for just a short while and let your body rest. What the meditation is attempting to do is help you to *connect* in a loving way to the people in your life that you come into contact with every day. It is equally important to connect in a loving way to ourselves! We so often ignore taking care of ourselves while we are busy taking care of others.

Loving-Kindness Meditation

> *May I be filled with loving kindness*
> *May I be well*
> *May I be peaceful and at ease*
> *May I be happy*

As you say this meditation, let the feelings arise with the words. Repeat the phrases over and over again, letting the feelings go all through your body and mind. This is a meditation that can help you connect to your heart and be aware of how to connect to others in a *heartful* way.

 # Credits

INTRODUCTION

Page 1: From *Credibility: How Leaders Gain and Lose It, Why People Demand It* by James M. Kouzes and Barry Z. Posner (p.30), copyright © 2003 by John Wiley & Sons, Inc. San Francisco: Jossey-Bass.

Page 4: From *The Blessings Already Are* by John Morton (p.12), copyright © 2000 by Peace Theological Seminary and College of Philosophy. Reprinted with permission of Mandeville Press.

CHAPTER 1

Page 20: From *Illusions: The Adventures of a Reluctant Messiah* by Richard Bach (p.169), copyright © 1977 by Richard Bach and Leslie Parrish-Bach. Used by permission of Dell Publishing, a division of Random House, Inc.

CHAPTER 2

Page 27: From *Encouraging the Heart: A Leader's Guide to Rewarding and Recognizing Others* by James M. Kouzes and Barry Z. Posner (pp.58-59), copyright © 1999 by John Wiley & Sons, Inc. Reprinted with permission of John Wiley & Sons, Inc.

Page 32: From *Rethinking Alzheimer's Care* by Sam Fazio, Dorothy Seman, and Jane Stansell (p.95). Reprinted with permission of Health Professions Press, Inc.

CHAPTER 3

Page 39: Two excerpts from *The Path of Blessing: Experiencing the Energy and Abundance of the Divine* by Marcia Prager (cover & p.4), copyright © 1998 by Marcia Prager (2003 first Jewish Lights Publishing). Permission granted by Jewish Lights Publishing, P.O. Box 237, Woodstock, VT 05091, www.jewishlights.com.

Page 44: From *My Grandfather's Blessings: Stories of Strength, Refuge and Belonging* by Rachel Naomi Remen, M.D. (p.214), copyright © 2000 by Rachel Naomi Remen, M.D. Used by permission of Riverhead Books, an imprint of Penguin Group (USA), Inc.

CHAPTER 9

Pages 119, 123, 131: From *From Beginning to End: The Rituals of Our Lives* by Robert Fulghum (pp.19 & 25), copyright © 1995 by Robert Fulghum. Published by Ballantine Books, a division of Random House Books, Inc.

Page 126: From *Encouraging the Heart: A Leader's Guide to Rewarding and Recognizing Others* by James M. Kouzes and Barry Z. Posner (p.123), copyright © 1999 by John Wiley & Sons, Inc. Reprinted with permission of John Wiley & Sons, Inc.

Page 127: From *Rituals for Our Times: Celebrating, Healing, and Changing Our Lives and Our Relationships* by Evan Imber-Black and Janine Roberts. Copyright © 1998. Used with permission of Jason Aronson, an imprint of Rowman & Littlefield Publishers, Inc.

CHAPTER 10

Pages 133, 143: (Meir) From *God Is at Eye Level* by Jan Pillips (p.142). Copyright © 2000 by Jan Phillips (p.142). Used with permission of Quest Books, www.questbooks.net.

Page 133: From *You Learn by Living: Eleven Keys for a More Fulfilling Life* by Eleanor Roosevelt. Copyright © 1983. Louisville, KY: Westminster John Knox Press.

Pages 138, 143: From *A Tiny Treasury of African Proverbs* by Ariel. Copyright © 1998. Kansas City, MO: Andrews McMeel Publishing.

CHAPTER 11

Page 149: From *The Little Prince* by Antoine de Saint-Exupery (p.63), English translation copyright © 1943 by Harcourt, Inc. and renewed 1971 by Consuelo de Saint-Exupery, English translation copyright © 2000 by Richard Howard. Reprinted by permission of Harcourt, Inc.

Pages 152, 157: From *Zen Mind, Beginner's Mind* by Shunryu Suzuki Roshi, copyright © 1973. New York: Weatherhill.

Page 155: (Mansfield) From *God Is at Eye Level* by Jan Pillips (p.14). Copyright © 2000 by Jan Phillips. Used with permission of Quest Books, www.questbooks.net.

CHAPTER 12

Pages 159, 169: From *Kitchen Table Wisdom: Stories that Heal* by Rachel Naomi Remen, M.D. (p.143), copyright © 1996 by Rachel Naomi Remen, M.D. Used by permission of Riverhead Books, an imprint of Penguin Group (USA), Inc.

Pages 164, 170: From *The Dance: Moving to the Rhythms of Your True Self* by Oriah Mountain Dreamer (p.154), copyright © 2001 by Oriah Mountain Dreamer. Reprinted with permission of HarperCollins Publishers, Inc.

CHAPTER 13

Page 173: From *My Grandfather's Blessings: Stories of Strength, Refuge and Belonging* by Rachel Naomi Remen, M.D. (p.2), copyright © 2000 by Rachel Naomi Remen, M.D. Used by permission of Riverhead Books, an imprint of Penguin Group (USA), Inc.

Page 174: (Meir) From *God Is at Eye Level* by Jan Pillips (p.142). Copyright © 2000 by Jan Phillips. Used with permission of Quest Books, www.questbooks.net.

Page 177: From *My Grandfather's Blessings: Stories of Strength, Refuge and Belonging* by Rachel Naomi Remen, M.D. (p.280), copyright © 2000 by Rachel Naomi Remen, M.D. Used by permission of Riverhead Books, an imprint of Penguin Group (USA), Inc.

CHAPTER 14

Page 187: From *The Soul Would Have No Rainbow if the Eyes Had No Tears* by Guy Zona, copyright © 1994. Touchstone Books.

Page 187: From *My Grandfather's Blessings: Stories of Strength, Refuge and Belonging* by Rachel Naomi Remen, M.D. (p.303), copyright © 2000 by Rachel Naomi Remen, M.D. Used by permission of Riverhead Books, an imprint of Penguin Group (USA), Inc.

Page 188: From *The Prophet* by Kahlil Gibran, copyright © 1923. New York: Knopf Publishing Group, a division of Random House, Inc.

Page 191: From *Living a Life that Matters* by Harold S. Kushner (p.154), copyright © 2001 by Harold S. Kushner. Used with permission of Anchor Books, an imprint of Random House, Inc.

Page 193: From *Still Here* by Ram Dass (p.131), copyright © 2000 by Ram Dass. Used by permission of Riverhead Books, an imprint of Penguin Group (USA) Inc.

Page 193: From *A Path with Heart: A Guide Through the Perils and Promises of Spiritual Life* by Jack Kornfield (p.16), copyright © 1993 by Jack Kornfield. Reprinted with permission of Bantam Books, a division of Random House, Inc.

Page 195: From *Still Here* by Ram Dass (pp.24-25), copyright © 2000 by Ram Dass. Used by permission of Riverhead Books, an imprint of Penguin Group (USA) Inc.

Page 196: From *The Soul Would Have No Rainbow if the Eyes Had No Tears* by Guy Zona, copyright © 1994. Touchstone Books.

Page 196: From *The Prophet* by Kahlil Gibran (p.29), copyright © 1923. New York: Knopf Publishing Group, a division of Random House, Inc.